MAJOR PROBLEMS IN INTERNAL MEDICINE

Published

Cline: Cancer Chemotherapy (second edition by Cline and Haskell
  now available separately)
Shearn: Sjögren's Syndrome
Cogan: Ophthalmic Manifestations of Systemic Vascular Disease
Williams: Rheumatoid Arthritis as a Systemic Disease
Cluff, Caranasos and Stewart: Clinical Problems with Drugs
Fries and Holman: Systemic Lupus Erythematosus
Kass: Pernicious Anemia
Braude: Antimicrobial Drug Therapy
Bray: The Obese Patient
Zieve and Levin: Bleeding Disorders
Gorlin: Coronary Artery Disease
Bunn, Forget and Ranney: Hemoglobinopathies
Sleisenger and Brandborg: Malabsorption
Beeson and Bass: The Eosinophil
Krugman and Gocke: Viral Hepatitis
Hurwitz, Duranceau, and Haddad: Disorders of Esophageal Motility
Galambos: Cirrhosis
Nelson: The Adrenal Cortex: Physiological Function and Disease
Raskin and Appenzeller: Headache

MAJOR PROBLEMS IN INTERNAL MEDICINE

In Preparation

Potts: Disorders of Calcium Metabolism
Havel and Kane: Diagnosis and Treatment of Hyperlipidemias
Siltzbach: Sarcoidosis
Scheinberg and Sternlieb: Wilson's Disease and Copper Metabolism
Atkins and Bodel: Fever
Lieber and De Carli: Medical Aspects of Alcoholism
Merrill: Glomerulonephritis
Goldberg: The Scientific Basis and Practical Use of Diuretics
Kilbourne: Influenza
Deykin: Diseases of the Platelets
Cohen: Amyloidosis
Salmon: Multiple Myeloma
Weinstein: Infective Endocarditis
Sasahara: Pulmonary Embolism
Smith: Renal Lithiasis
Swartz: Meningitis
Sparling: Venereal Diseases
McLees: Critical Care
Engel: Psychosocial Problems in Medical Practice
Utz: Systemic Mycotic Infections
Solomon and Chopra: Graves Disease and Hyperthyroidism

FRANK P. BROOKS, M.D., Sc.D. (Med)
Professor of Medicine and Physiology;
Hospital of the University of Pennsylvania,
Philadelphia, Pennsylvania

DISEASES OF THE EXOCRINE PANCREAS

VOLUME

XX

IN THE SERIES

MAJOR PROBLEMS IN INTERNAL MEDICINE

Lloyd H. Smith, Jr., M.D., *Editor*

W. B. SAUNDERS COMPANY • PHILADELPHIA • LONDON • TORONTO 1980

W. B. Saunders Company: West Washington Square
Philadelphia, PA   19105

1 St. Anne's Road
Eastbourne, East Sussex BN21, 3UN, England

1 Goldthorne Avenue
Toronto, Ontario M8Z 5T9, Canada

Library of Congress Cataloging in Publication Data

Brooks, Frank P   1920–

Diseases of the exocrine pancreas.

(Major problems in internal medicine ; v. 20)

1.   Pancreas—Diseases.   I. Title.   II. Series.
    [DNLM: 1.   Pancreatic diseases. W1 MA492T v. 20 /
    WI800 B873d]

RC 857.B76   616.3'7   79-67788

ISBN   0-7216-2077-9

Diseases of the Exocrine Pancreas   ISBN   0-7216-2077-9

Last digit is the print number: 9   8   7   6   5   4   3   2   1

To Professor J. Earl Thomas — distinguished physiologist,
superb experimentalist, memorable teacher and friend.

FOREWORD

The pancreas was long an obscure organ tucked away in the posterior abdomen. Vesalius considered it to be only a support for the stomach, and in the Talmud it was termed "the finger of the liver." It remains perversely difficult to study by physical examination, radiologic techniques, biopsy or analysis of physiologic function. Despite this perversity, the pancreas deserves respect for its importance and versatility in metabolism, nutrition and endocrinology. Trypsin was the first isolated protein to be termed an enzyme, and secretin was the first defined hormone. Many of the basic studies on the cell physiology of protein synthesis, packaging and secretion as zymogen granules were carried out on pancreatic acinar cells. The islets have continued to be fertile sites for endocrine research for more than half a century.

Why are the islets scattered throughout the substance of the exocrine pancreas? Is there any rationale for having a million small endocrine packets peppered randomly about an organ that is otherwise resolutely dedicated to facilitating intraluminal digestion? Why should there be apposition of the cells that secrete insulin and glucagon (and gastrin, vasoactive intestinal polypeptide and other products) to the clustered acinar cells that are programmed to secrete amylase, lipase and a variety of proteases? No clear answer to these questions has been obtained, and perhaps we should not strain teleology too far. The pancreas may represent only a marriage of anatomic convenience for its endocrine and exocrine components.

Disease of the islets has attracted great attention in internal medicine since 1886, when Minkowski and Von Mering produced experimental diabetes in the dog by total pancreatectomy. The study of the various syndromes of diabetes mellitus has continued ever since but with much yet to learn about the interplay of such variables as genetics, viral infections and immunology. Other syndromes of hormone excess have been described for insulin, glucagon, gastrin and vasoactive intestinal polypeptide. This "islet work" has had virtually no relationship to "acinar work," carried out by different investigators in different laboratories in different medical disciplines.

The exocrine pancreas is relatively inaccessible to the internist, but unfortunately it is not infrequently the site of serious illness. For the internist its most important illnesses are pancreatitis (acute and chronic) and carcinoma. Pancreatitis remains a mysterious disorder with overtones of autoinjury presumably set in motion by a wide variety of inciting agents — alcohol, other drugs, excess ionized calcium or lipids, biliary tract disease, trauma and even heredity. Both diagnosis and therapy are nonspecific. As noted in this monograph, carcinoma of the pancreas seems to be increasing in frequency in a pattern that is the obverse of the decline of carcinoma of the stomach. It now accounts for 5 per cent of all cancer deaths in the United States. Almost invariably the diagnosis is made late and the prognosis is very poor. In fact, no increase in survival for patients with pancreatic adenocarcinoma has been obtained over the last three decades.

In this monograph, *Diseases of the Exocrine Pancreas,* Dr. Frank P. Brooks has furnished a scholarly review of pancreatic function in health and disease, with major emphasis on clinical factors of importance to the practicing internist. The individual chapters summarize the current state of knowledge about the pathogenesis, clinical presentation, diagnosis, therapy and prognosis of acute pancreatitis, chronic pancreatitis, chronic relapsing pancreatitis, carcinoma and other tumors of the exocrine pancreas and cystic fibrosis. The monograph is supplemented with an excellent and up-to-date bibliography about these disorders concerning which there is still much controversy. This summary, based on Dr. Brooks's extensive personal experience at the Hospital of the University of Pennsylvania and his review of the published experience of others, is an important contribution to the literature of internal medicine.

Lloyd H. Smith, Jr., M.D.

ACKNOWLEDGMENTS

The assistance of Mrs. Mary Jane Payne and the secretarial staff of the Gastrointestinal Section of the Department of Medicine, Hospital of the University of Pennsylvania, is gratefully acknowledged.

FRANK P. BROOKS, M.D.

CONTENTS

CHAPTER 1

INTRODUCTION

Diseases of the Exocrine Pancreas is addressed to the general internist in an attempt to improve the diagnosis and management of pancreatic disease by this important group of primary care physicians. It is divided into two main sections: clinical problems and basic science considerations. The section on clinical problems is subdivided into four main chapters: Acute Pancreatitis; Chronic Pancreatitis; Carcinoma of the Pancreas; and Cystic Fibrosis. Each chapter is divided into 12 parts: (1) how the patient presents; (2) risk factors in diagnosis; (3) laboratory diagnosis; (4) diagnosis and differential diagnosis; (5) clinical course; (6) treatment; (7) epidemiology; (8) pathophysiology; (9) animal models; (10) etiology; (11) screening; and (12) prevention. The section on basic science presents a brief overview of pancreatic physiology.

Acute pancreatitis is responsible for about the same number of age-adjusted deaths as acute appendicitis in the United States. Chronic pancreatitis occurs in about one third as many patients as acute pancreatitis.[2] The distinction between multiple attacks of acute pancreatitis and recurrent chronic pancreatitis (chronic relapsing pancreatitis) is uncertain, however (Fig. 1–1). Theoretically, in the former, the pancreas should return to an entirely normal state between attacks, but our ability to detect minimal pancreatic damage does not allow us to make the distinction. Chronic pancreatitis with insufficiency is characterized by excessive fat in the stool resulting from inability to digest dietary fat. This represents the end stage of chronic pancreatitis. Some patients have pancreatic insufficiency with little histopathologic evidence of inflammation. It is a situation similar to the distinction between atrophic gastritis and gastric atrophy. It is likely that such pancreatic insufficiency is a later stage in the evolution of chronic pancreatitis in some patients.

Cancer of the pancreas is increasing in incidence in the United States, almost in a parallel course with the decrease in incidence of cancer of the stomach. It is now the fourth most common death-causing cancer in man in this country. About 98 to 99 per cent of pancreatic cancers are fatal.

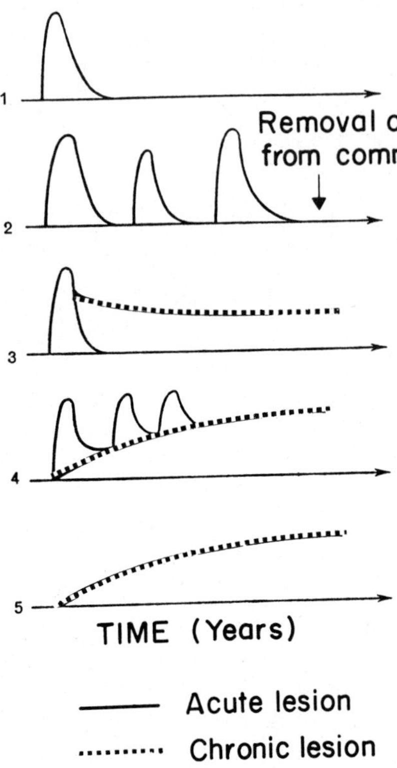

Figure 1-1. Diagrammatic representation of the clinical course of pancreatitis in relation to the inflammatory lesion in the pancreas. (Modified from Benhamou, J. P., and Sarles, H.: Foie, pancréas, voies biliaires. Paris, Flammarion, 1972, p. 121.)

Cystic fibrosis is the most common genetic disease of the digestive tract in the United States, occurring about once in every 2000 live births. Although formerly it was almost exclusively a disease of children, successful treatment, particularly of its respiratory complications, has resulted in survival into adult life of an increasing number of patients.

The general internist can therefore expect to see pancreatic disease among his or her patients. The author's experience suggests that often the generalist's index of suspicion is low, and that excessive reliance is placed upon the serum amylase level in the diagnosis of pancreatitis. A number of new diagnostic techniques are developing that will be available to the internist, and a more rational basis for treatment now exists. I shall attempt to emphasize these considerations in the following pages.

REFERENCES

1. Mendeloff, A. I., and Dunn, J. P.: Digestive Diseases. Cambridge, Harvard University Press, 1971, pp. 105–113
2. O'Sullivan, J. N., Nobrega, F. T., Morlock, C. G., Brown, A. L., Jr., and Bartholomew, L. G.: Acute and chronic pancreatitis in Rochester, Minn., 1940–1969. Gastroenterology 62:373–379, 1972

SECTION I
CLINICAL PROBLEMS

CHAPTER 2

ACUTE PANCREATITIS

HOW THE PATIENT WITH ACUTE PANCREATITIS PRESENTS

The most common complaint of the patient with acute pancreatitis is pain (Table 2–1). It may be the sudden onset of excruciatingly severe pain or a more gradual onset of moderate abdominal pain several hours after a large meal. There is some degree of localization of pain within the pancreas. Painful stimuli in the head of the pancreas are perceived as pain in the right upper quadrant; those in the body, in the epigastrium; and those in the tail, in the left upper quadrant. In acute pancreatitis the pain is localized to the epigastrium in about two thirds of the patients, whereas in most of the others the pain is diffuse and difficult to localize. About one third of patients report that the pain radiates to the back. The pain is usually continuous for periods of hours, and only infrequently (15 per cent of patients) is it intermittent in character. The pain is probably due to inflammation, with stimulation of nerve endings, and to swelling of the gland, with increased tension on the capsule.[112, 162] Obstruction of pancreatic ducts is also a factor.[112] Recently, sublingual nitroglycerin was found to relieve severe pancreatic pain promptly after endoscopic retrograde cholangiopancreatography (ERCP), suggesting a role of vascular factors in pancreatic pain.[173]

Pain is absent in only 1 to 2 per cent of patients with acute pancreatitis. Some of these patients present in shock. In recurrent acute pancreatitis in patients who abuse alcohol, pain is still the most common symptom, but its character and severity are more variable. In some patients the pain may be relatively mild but is usually worse after eating. In others, a boring quality of the pain with radiation to the back may be prominent. Antacids are rarely helpful in relieving the

*TABLE 2–1.　SYMPTOMS AND SIGNS IN PATIENTS WITH
ACUTE PANCREATITIS*

Abdominal pain	93–97%
Nausea and vomiting	30–90%
Shock	25–60%
Mental confusion	27%
Pleural effusion	8–25%
Abdominal distention	7–80%
Ileus	50–80%
Fever	60–95%
Jaundice	9–30%
Ascites	2

pain. Salicylates may be of use early in the course, but all too often patients find that codeine, meperidine (Demerol) or opiates are necessary, and addiction follows. Localization of the pain to the abdominal wall may occur with the formation of pseudocysts or a pancreatic abscess. Characteristically, the pain is out of proportion to the physical findings.[9]

Since abdominal pain is common to many abdominal disorders, it is of critical importance to integrate the history with the findings on physical examination of the abdomen. In acute pancreatitis there is characteristically diffuse abdominal tenderness, without localized signs of peritoneal irritation such as localized tenderness, muscle spasm or rebound tenderness. Sometimes a poorly defined mass may be palpated. This may represent an edematous, inflamed pancreas, omentum involved in the inflammatory process or a pseudocyst.[41] A decision to perform a laparotomy depends upon the evaluation of the physical signs in the abdomen suggesting a perforated viscus or localized inflammatory disease such as cholecystitis or appendicitis. Table 2–2 lists some diseases producing abdominal pain that must be considered in the differential diagnosis of acute pancreatitis.

TABLE 2–2.　DIFFERENTIAL DIAGNOSIS OF ACUTE PANCREATITIS

1. Perforated peptic ulcer
2. Acute cholecystitis
3. Perforated gastric carcinoma
4. Acute appendicitis
5. Ruptured spleen
6. Liver abscess
7. Alcoholic hepatitis
8. Acute porphyria
9. Perinephric abscess
10. Myocardial infarction
11. Mesenteric thrombosis or embolism
12. Ischemic colitis

Nausea and vomiting can be expected in 30 to 90 per cent of patients with acute pancreatitis. The vomitus is usually gastric content but may contain bile. The amount is usually no more than 200 to 300 ml. The amount of vomitus may be much greater if a pseudocyst forms and compresses the gastric outlet, simulating pyloric obstruction. Hematemesis occurs in only 1 to 2 per cent of patients with acute pancreatitis. It may be the result of acute gastric erosions or a tear at the esophagogastric junction (Mallory-Weiss syndrome). Rarely, pancreatic pseudocysts may produce portal hypertension, leading to esophageal varices and hematemesis.[211]

Shock is often the presenting feature of acute hemorrhagic pancreatitis without pain.[205] Among one group of fatal cases, more than 30 per cent died in shock during the first week of the disease, and another 12 per cent later on.[195] Shock and coma are commonly dominant features in patients in whom the diagnosis of acute pancreatitis was unsuspected until autopsy.[224] Hypertension may be present in as many as 40 per cent of patients with acute pancreatitis.[157] Mental confusion was present in 27 per cent of 100 patients in one prospective study.[157] Agitation is also common.[9]

Pleural effusions or areas of atelectasis above the diaphragm, especially on the left side, are present in up to 25 per cent of patients with acute pancreatitis.[157] A chest roentgenogram will occasionally provide the first clue to the nature of the intra-abdominal disease. Abdominal distention is a common feature of acute pancreatitis. It is usually the result of ileus.[157] Rarely, mechanical obstruction can occur late in the course of acute pancreatitis owing to intestinal stenosis secondary to ischemia.

Fever is present in most patients with acute pancreatitis. Persistent temperature elevation suggests a complication. Jaundice is present in about 10 per cent of patients with acute pancreatitis. It may be due to inflammation from pancreatitis around the common duct rather than common duct stones in a third of patients with common duct obstruction.[27] Medical causes such as cirrhosis accounted for jaundice in more than half the patients coming to autopsy.[61]

Pancreatic ascites is an unusual finding but seems to have been noted more commonly in recent years. It is due to rupture of a pancreatic duct proximal to a site of obstruction. More than half the patients with ascites have pseudocysts.

A number of other findings occur rarely but are sufficiently dramatic to be worth recalling even though they are not specific. These include ecchymoses in the flanks (Grey-Turner's sign), occurring in 1 per cent of patients, periumbilical ecchymoses (Cullen's sign), occurring in 1 per cent, and multiple painful necrotic skin nodules resembling erythema nodosum due to fat necrosis.[95, 145]

TABLE 2–3. RISK FACTORS IN ACUTE PANCREATITIS

1. Alcohol abuse
2. Gallstones
3. Abdominal trauma
4. Infections: mumps, other viruses
5. Ischemic vascular disease
6. Hyperlipidemias
7. Hyperparathyroidism
8. Drugs: steroids, diuretics, immunosuppressives
9. Duodenal disease: periampullary diverticula, Crohn's disease
10. Postoperative state, especially after gastrectomy
11. Immunologic disorders
12. Cancer of the pancreas
13. Pancreatitis of pregnancy
14. Acute intermittent porphyria

RISK FACTORS IN THE DIAGNOSIS OF ACUTE PANCREATITIS

An important consideration in making the diagnosis of acute pancreatitis is the recognition of factors known to be associated with an increased risk of developing the disease. Table 2–3 lists these factors. The presence of any of them should alert the physician to the possibility of pancreatitis as the cause of abdominal disease. In some hospitals, the last decade has seen a dramatic shift from gallstones to alcohol abuse as the most common risk factor in acute pancreatitis.[100, 195] In large municipal hospitals and Veterans Administration hospitals, the great majority of patients with pancreatitis are also abusers of alcohol. Some students of pancreatitis believe that acute pancreatitis in an alcoholic always develops in an already damaged pancreas, but subtle injuries to the pancreas cannot be detected with any simpler means than biopsy.

In nonalcoholic patients, gallstones remain the most common risk factor in acute pancreatitis.[93, 95] Recent reports indicate that finding gallstones in the feces by straining the stool after daily enemas for 10 days is a very accurate method of detecting gallstone pancreatitis. Gallstones were recovered in 92 per cent of 51 patients with gallstone pancreatitis. Single and, in about a third of the patients, multiple stones were passed within the first 10 days after the onset of symptoms. Only 6 of 51 patients with gallstones but without pancreatitis passed stones in their feces. No stones were found in the stools of 10 patients with alcoholic pancreatitis or in those of 12 patients with stenosing papillitis.[3, 4]

Abdominal trauma, especially after auto accidents in which the steering wheel compresses the abdomen, has become an important cause of pancreatitis.[81] Contusions, lacerations and transections of the ducts of the pancreas are the major types of injury. Fistulas are common during the first 4 weeks but they usually heal. Pseudocysts develop in 2 to 10 per cent of patients with pancreatic trauma, and another 3 per cent develop persistent or recurrent pancreatitis.[153, 203] In various reports of acute pancreatitis, trauma accounted for the pancreatitis in 1 to 18 per cent of patients, with an average of 5 per cent. It is the most common cause of acute pancreatitis in children.[136]

The evidence for infections as a cause of acute pancreatitis rests largely on rises in blood agglutinin or precipitin titers after the onset of the disease. Viral infections have been suspect, with mumps as a prime example. Elevations of both serum amylase and serum lipase in patients with mumps and abdominal pain have led to an estimate that about 2 per cent of patients with mumps develop pancreatitis.[92] More recently, infections with Coxsackie B viruses and *Mycoplasma pneumoniae* have been associated with acute pancreatitis.[13, 31, 59, 92] About 4 per cent of a large series of patients had a significant rise in antibody titer against a number of viruses between the first and second weeks after the onset of pancreatitis.[13]

Ischemic vascular disease is implicated as a factor in less than 10 per cent of all patients with acute pancreatitis, and in most cases the patients are over the age of 70 and have other manifestations of vascular disease. Only rarely is the diagnosis made in life. Atheromatous embolization from plaques in the aorta to the pancreas is more frequent than would be expected by chance alone but the mechanism is still unclear.

Abdominal pain may be associated with hyperlipidemia without other evidence of pancreatic disease. Sufficient data have been published, however, to indicate that patients with hyperlipidemia of Types I, IV and V are at increased risk for the development of pancreatitis.[71, 88] Hyperlipidemia appears to be a more important factor in the pancreatitis of young persons who are not abusers of alcohol. Because serum lipids may be elevated acutely in pancreatitis due to alcohol and other causes (3 to 20 per cent), levels should be determined again during convalescence.[30, 42, 56] Some authors have found an incidence of pancreatitis as high as 50 per cent in patients with Types I, IV and V hyperlipidemia, but the criteria for the diagnosis of pancreatitis in these patients leave much to be desired.[107]

Patients with hyperparathyroidism have an increased risk of developing acute pancreatitis. The incidence of the disease among these patients is estimated at 6 to 12 per cent, which is significantly higher than that among the general population.[210] On the other hand, primary hyperparathyroidism accounts for less than 1 per cent of all cases of acute pancreatitis.

A wide variety of drugs have been implicated as causes of acute pancreatitis, largely on the basis of case reports of patients developing acute pancreatitis while receiving the drug. The list of drugs includes corticosteroids, thiazide diuretics and oral contraceptives.[32, 133] More recently furosemide, azathioprine and paracetamol (Tylenol) have been added.[70] It would seem prudent to obtain a careful history of medications taken by the patient, with particular reference to those mentioned as potential causes of pancreatitis.

Abnormalities in the duodenum that might predispose to partial obstruction of, or to reflux of intestinal content into, the pancreatic duct are logical risk factors in acute pancreatitis. Crohn's disease of the duodenum is a recognized but rare cause of acute pancreatitis. Gastroenterologists performing ERCP have been impressed with periampullary duodenal diverticula as factors in pancreatitis, but the exact incidence is difficult to determine.[147]

Postoperative pancreatitis is a dreaded complication of gastric and biliary tract surgery.[166, 167] The criteria for diagnosis short of re-exploration or autopsy are still unsatisfactory. Certainly many postoperative patients are found to have elevated serum amylase levels without clinical signs of pancreatitis. Among those in whom the full clinical syndrome appears, the mortality may reach more than 40 per cent. Surgery involving the gastrointestinal tract and coincident biliary tract disease account for more than three fourths of the cases, with gastrectomy the major offender.[167]

The role of abnormal immune reactions and hypersensitivity as factors in acute pancreatitis is very uncertain. Acute pancreatitis does occur in certain diseases considered to involve "autoimmune" phenomena, such as lupus erythematosus, Sjögren's syndrome and rheumatoid arthritis. Antibodies to pancreatic tissue have been found in the blood of patients with pancreatitis.[118] As with other antibodies, it is difficult to distinguish between causative and secondary roles. Patients with malignant hypertension and renal failure have an increased risk of acute pancreatitis.[16]

Recent studies have reported that acute pancreatitis complicates renal transplantation in about 3 to 6 per cent of patients.[38, 165, 177, 198, 204] All patients were receiving steroids and azathioprine. The fatality rate was nearly 50 per cent. Acute pancreatitis occurs in patients with fulminant hepatic failure as a terminal and often unsuspected event.[83, 154, 164, 215] These patients also usually receive steroids and sometimes azathioprine, but in those cases secondary to viral hepatitis the virus itself may play a role. Again, the mortality rate is high. Acute pancreatitis can complicate both primary and metastatic carcinoma of the pancreas.[63, 151] Histologic evidence of pancreatitis may be present in 10 per cent of patients with carcinoma of the pancreas, but in one study only 2 per cent had clinical evidence of pancreatitis.[63] Acute pancreatitis can occur during pregnancy, usually in the last trimester or immediately post partum. Gallstones are present in some patients. Hyperlipidemia may contribute in some uncertain way. Finally, acute intermittent porphyria has occurred coincidentally with acute pancreatitis and greatly complicated the interpretation of abdominal pain.

After considering all these risk factors, it should be admitted that there remain a number of patients with acute pancreatitis who do not have any recognizable predisposing factors to account for their disease. The proportion of these patients ranges from 10 to 30 per cent in various series.

LABORATORY DIAGNOSIS OF ACUTE PANCREATITIS

The diagnosis of acute pancreatitis depends primarily upon the history and physical examination. The recognition of risk factors and a high index of suspicion are very important. Since none of these findings are specific for pancreatitis, the prudent physician will use selected laboratory tests to confirm clinical impressions and reinforce risk factors in raising the suspicion of acute pancreatitis. By far the most widely used laboratory test is the estimation of amylase activity — in blood, urine or peritoneal fluid.[181]

Amylase Determinations

The standard techniques of amylase determination are the saccharogenic, iodometric and chromogenic methods. Saccharogenic methods are based upon the digestion of a starch substrate and the determination of the amount of sugar (reducing substances) produced. Results are usually reported in Somogyi units. The iodometric methods are based upon the reaction of iodine with the products of starch digestion, producing colored substances. The chromogenic method involves coupling a dye with starch to form a substrate. When the combination is exposed to amylase, the dye is split off, and a color reaction can be used to detect the end product. Fortunately for physicians' memories the normal values of serum amylase activity by either the saccharogenic or the chromogenic methods are numerically similar (40 to 180 units). Most patients with serum amylase values over 1000 have pancreatic disease. Many patients with acute pancreatitis have values in the normal range or up to 300 units, however.[2] The reasons for this are not completely understood but include the fact that pancreatic amylase is quickly cleared into the urine by the kidneys. Hyperlipidemia may suppress elevation of amylase activity determined by iodometric methods in patients with acute pancreatitis.[55] The presence of an elevated serum amylase is most dependable in acute pancreatitis when the determination is performed within 48 hours of the onset of symptoms. Elevated amylase levels in the urine of patients with acute pancreatitis persist for longer periods of time. It appears to be characteristic of acute pancreatitis that the renal tubular reabsorption of amylase (and other small proteins) is significantly decreased. As in the case of the serum amylase, urine amylase outputs of more than 1000 units per hour usually indicate pancreatic disease. The normal level is up to 300 units, however, and increased levels in the zone of 300 to 1000 units are less specific.[64, 187, 216] Urine should be collected for 2 to 3 hours and expressed as output units per hour.[214] Collections for 12 to 24 hours are often impractical and do not add substantially to the diagnostic value of the test.

The problem of an elevated serum amylase after a laparotomy can be a source of considerable concern.[34] Among 100 consecutive patients having upper abdominal surgery, 6 had serum amylase levels of greater than 150 units 24 hours later. Four of these patients had had a cholecystectomy. Only one had clinical evidence of pancreatitis.[139] In another series of 107 patients, 13 had elevated serum amylase levels postoperatively, and one died of acute pancreatitis.[102] Either pancreatic or nonpancreatic isoamylases may be elevated transiently in about 16 per cent of patients during the postoperative period.[86] In a study of patients with traumatic pancreatitis after blunt trauma to the abdomen, the serum amylase was elevated in about half. The urine amylase may serve as a guide to stopping nasogastric suction, since after penetrating abdominal injury only 1 per cent of patients had elevated serum amylase values.[225]

Among patients with diabetic ketoacidosis and abdominal pain, elevated values of serum amylase were found in 60 per cent of 35 episodes but probably did not indicate pancreatitis.[72, 108] Elevation of serum amylase occurs in chronic liver disease and may be due to a secondary pancreatic isoenzyme which does not appear in the urine.[218]

The relation of the severity of acute pancreatitis to the degree of elevation of serum amylase has been found to be unpredictable. Patients with fatal acute hemorrhagic pancreatitis whose serum amylase values were normal have been reported. There are two observations worthy of attention: (1) persistent elevations of the serum amylase for more than 3 weeks may indicate, in a patient with acute pancreatitis, the development of a pseudocyst;[89, 212] and (2) patients with gallstone-related acute pancreatitis, as opposed to acute alcoholic pancreatitis, tend to have higher values of serum amylase.[5, 119]

Table 2–4 shows data on the serum amylase in a number of other diseases.[80, 82, 128, 131] Again, the higher the serum amylase value, the more likely it is that pancreatic disease is present.[170] Opiates produce elevation of the serum amylase in some subjects.[23, 79]

Elevated levels of amylase in peritoneal fluid have been reported in acute pancreatitis and in "pancreatic ascites." It is difficult to determine how important the results are in the diagnosis and management of acute pancreatitis. The level of amylase in the peritoneal fluid should be substantially above that in the serum.[227] In pancreatic ascites values from 300 to several thousand units of amylase can be expected.[67] Pleural fluid in acute pancreatitis also contains amylase activity in excess of the serum levels.

Another problem in the use of serum amylase in the diagnosis of acute pancreatitis is the presence of serum macroamylases. These are due to the presence of a complex of amylase with a large serum protein that prevents filtration at the kidney glomerulus and results in elevated serum amylase values but low renal clearance of amylase. Up to 5 per cent of patients found to have elevated serum amylase have macroamylases. Some of these patients have pancreatic disease, but others have normal pancreatic function. Proof of the presence of a serum macroamylase can be obtained by rather simple methods, but these methods are still not widely available.

TABLE 2–4. *ELEVATIONS OF THE SERUM AMYLASE IN ACUTE PANCREATIC DISEASE AND NONPANCREATIC DISORDERS**[*]

	No. of Patients	%
Acute pancreatitis	42 of 42	100
	85 of 133	64
Peritonitis	9 of 13	69
Perforated peptic ulcer	8 of 51	6
	0 of 17	0
Peptic ulcer	18 of 112	6
Acute cholecystitis	7 of 75	10
Cholecystitis	21 of 119	18
Intestinal obstruction	4 of 20	20
Mesenteric thrombosis	2 of 6	33
Cirrhosis	0 of 17	0
	4 of 19	21
Renal disease	2 of 26	8
Chronic renal disease	0 of 32	0
Parotitis	13 of 15	87
Mumps	36 of 44	82
Opiates	6 of 27	22
	11 of 41	27
Diabetic ketoacidosis	8 of 10	80
	21 of 35	0
Upper abdominal surgery	10 of 107	12

[*]From Brooks, F. P., and Long, W. B.: Tests of pancreatic function. *In* Practice of Medicine, Vol. 11. Hagerstown, Md., Harper & Row, 1979.

TABLE 2–5. NORMAL SERUM AMYLASE VALUES (MG. GLUCOSE/DL.)*

AMYLASE	No. SUBJECTS	RANGE OF VALUES	P†	90% CONFIDENCE INTERVALS	
				Lower Limit	Upper Limit
Total	180	31–171	0.995	31–46	145–171
P-Type	122	14–96	0.98	14–18	64–96
S-Type	122	12–119	0.98	12–24	90–119

*From Heffernon, J. J., Fridhandler, L., Berk, J. E., and Shimamura, J.: Assay of amylase and isoamylase activities in serum and urine. Modifications in methods and range of normal values. Am. J. Gastroenterol. 67:474, 1977.

†Probability that range includes at least 95% of normal population.

As this chapter is being written exciting new developments are under way in the methodology of amylase determinations. It is now possible in the research laboratory to separate pancreatic from salivary amylase by chemical techniques.[19, 130] Table 2–5 shows normal values of each type. Note that the salivary amylase contributes a major portion of the normal total serum amylase activity. In acute pancreatitis, however, it is the pancreatic amylase that is elevated: the mean value in 51 patients was 51.0 units[19] (Table 2–6). The human pancreas may contain a salivary-type isoamylase.[188] Preliminary results indicate that these isoamylases can be separated by immunologic techniques as well. It is of interest that some patients with malignant tumors have elevated values of amylase in the serum as well as in the pleural and

TABLE 2–6. TOTAL AMYLASE AND ISOAMYLASE ACTIVITIES IN SERA FROM PATIENTS WITH ACUTE PANCREATITIS*

INITIALS	SEX	TOTAL	P	S	P/TOTAL × 100
T.L.B.	M	252	209	43	83.0
Pa. S.	M	1106	859	247	77.7
F.W.	F	828	734	94	88.6
D.W.	F	192	160	32	83.2
P.S.	F	1520	1383	137	91.0
			Mean		84.7
			SD		±5.22
			SE		±2.33

*The numbers represent units of reducing power generated per 100 ml. P is activity of pancreatic-type amylase, S is activity of salivary-type amylase.

From Fridhandler, L., Berk, J. E., and Ueda, M. Isolation and Measurement of pancreatic amylase in human sera and urine. Clin. Chemistry 18:1496, 1972.

peritoneal fluid. Thirty of 32 patients with carcinoma of the lung had elevated serum amylase.[20] It was usually a salivary amylase.[189] Both the primary tumor and metastases contained amylase. About 20 per cent of one group of heroin addicts had elevated serum amylase values, and most of these suffered from acute pulmonary disease.[87] About 15 per cent of 80 patients with lung disease also had elevated serum amylase values, mostly of the salivary type.[20, 187] A patient with elevated serum amylase was reported who had carcinoma of the ovary with elevated amylase activity in the tumor. The amylase was of the salivary type.[37] No tumor-associated isoenzymes have been identified consistently that would differentiate pancreatic from other carcinomas.[76] The cellular source and precise identification of the amylase under these circumstances remains to be determined.

Amylase-creatinine clearance ratio. The use of a ratio of amylase clearance to creatinine clearance was introduced in an attempt to improve the specificity and sensitivity of amylase determinations in acute pancreatitis. The calculation and normal values of amylase clearance in a large series of patients without pancreatic disease are shown in Table 2–7. Data from one of the original reports are reproduced in Figure 2–1.[125] On days 0–4 there is no overlap between patients with acute pancreatitis and healthy control subjects, but note that there is considerable overlap with "hospital controls," who constitute the real clinical problem. Initial reports emphasized the specificity and sensitivity of the amylase-creatinine clearance ratios in acute pancreatitis.[50, 146, 221] This was subsequently brought into question by reports of elevations occurring in patients with diabetic ketoacidosis and severe burns who did not have pancreatitis.[122] Others noted elevated values after thoracic surgery, including coronary bypass.[208] Patients with chronic renal insufficiency had ratios three

TABLE 2–7. C.A./C.C. RATIO*

Proposed upper limit normal range	200	1,200	4.0

$$\frac{C.A.}{C.C.} = \frac{\dfrac{[\text{Amylase}]_{\text{urine}} \times [\text{Volume}]_{\text{urine}}}{[\text{Amylase}]_{\text{serum}}} \times \text{Time}}{\dfrac{[\text{Creatinine}]_{\text{urine}} \times [\text{Volume}]_{\text{urine}}}{[\text{Creatinine}]_{\text{serum}}} \times \text{Time}}$$

$$\frac{C.A.}{C.C.}\% = \frac{[\text{Amylase}]_{\text{urine}} \times [\text{Creatinine}]_{\text{serum}}}{[\text{Amylase}]_{\text{serum}} \times [\text{Creatinine}]_{\text{urine}}} \times 100$$

*From Dreiling, D. A., Leichtling, J. J., and Janowitz, H. D.: The amylase-creatinine clearance ratio. Am. J. Gastroenterol. 61:291, 1974.

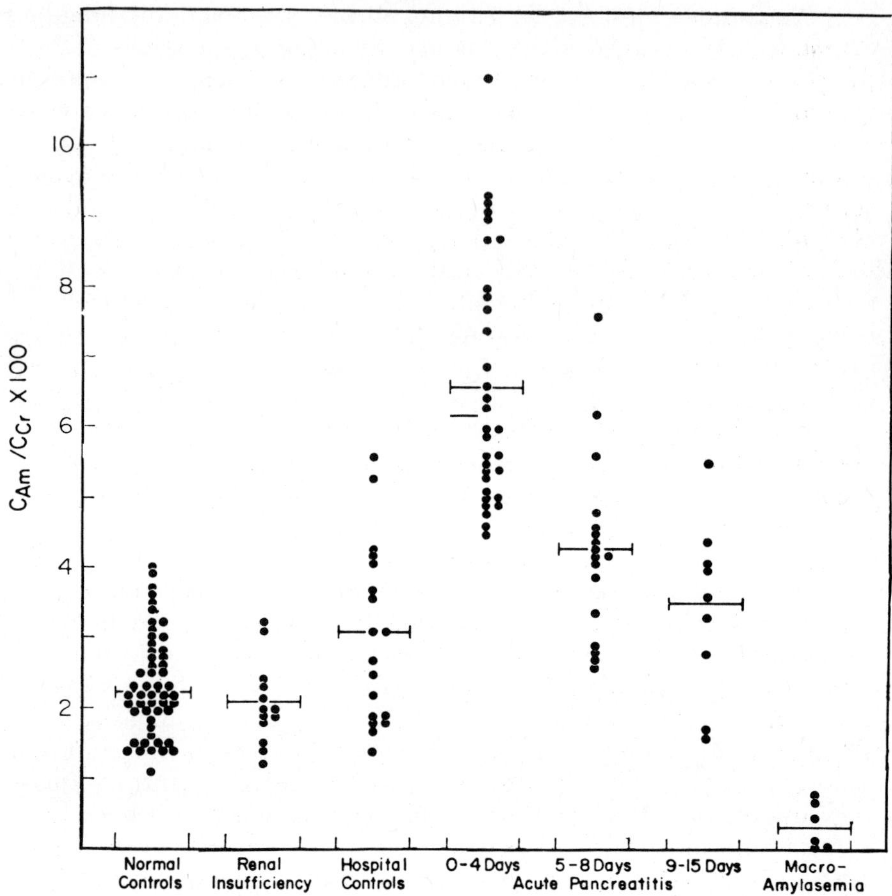

Figure 2–1. Amylase-creatinine clearance ratios in patients with acute pancreatitis, renal insufficiency, and macroamylasemia and in control subjects. (From Levitt, M. D., Rapoport, M., and Cooperband, S. R.: The renal clearance of amylase in renal insufficiency, acute pancreatitis and macroamylasemia. Ann. Intern. Med. 71:921, 1969.)

times those of controls, but a normal ratio did not exclude pancreatitis in patients on hemodialysis.[114, 142] In the patients with chronic renal insufficiency, the major component of the serum amylase was a pancreatic isoamylase.[105]

Normal ratios have been reported in a third of patients with acute pancreatitis even when the serum amylase was elevated.[114] Patients with biliary tract disease subjected to common duct exploration had elevated ratios in seven of eight instances in the absence of other evidence of acute pancreatitis.[46]

Technical problems, including the method used for measuring amylase, influence the results,[124] and hyperlipemia may reduce apparent amylase activity.[120, 219] Isoamylase measurements showed much higher clearance ratios of pancreatic amylase than of salivary amylase to creatinine in acute pancreatitis,[222] but an overlap between normal subjects and patients with acute pancreatitis remained.[128] It is generally agreed that the increased clearance ratio in acute pancreatitis is due to decreased renal tubular reabsorption of amylase by the kidney.[98, 217] In addition, other proteins such as microglobulins are cleared more rapidly.[123] Elevated glucagon levels do not account entirely for this.[134, 201] Proteinuria in myeloma and light chain proteinuria is also associated with increased clearance ratios. In the presence of macroamylasemia, the ratio of amylase to creatinine clearance should be normal.

At present, the physician entertaining a diagnosis of acute pancreatitis should obtain both serum and urine amylase determinations as early as possible in the course of the disease. Significant elevations suggest that acute pancreatitis is present, but the diagnosis should not be excluded by normal values if the clinical course is strongly suggestive. The value of the amylase-creatinine clearance ratio in acute pancreatitis must be considered uncertain.[123]

Other Laboratory Studies

Since the amylase activity has been found to be so variable, attention has been directed to other pancreatic enzymes. In general, serum lipase activity seems to parallel serum amylase activity.[126] It is not yet proven that in acute pancreatitis the serum lipase remains elevated longer than the serum amylase, but it does provide an independent assessment of exocrine-endocrine reflux. Recent studies indicate that the normal serum lipase is not of pancreatic origin but that after ERCP and injection of the ducts elevations in pancreatic lipase occur. In 44 young military personnel with mumps, the serum amylase was elevated in 82 per cent and the lipase in 8 of 11 patients tested.[216] A radioimmunoassay for trypsin or trypsinogen in the blood has been used with encouraging results in a small number of patients with acute pancreatitis.[202]

Other clinical laboratory tests may be useful in supporting the diagnosis or suggesting alternate diagnoses. The white blood cell count is usually elevated (10,000 to 30,000 per cu mm). Hypocalcemia is present in many patients and appears to correlate with the severity of the disease. Calcium values below 7 mg/100 ml indicate a poor prognosis. The lowest value usually occurs 5 to 7 days after the onset of symptoms. It is reasonable to expect that the hypocalcemia could be

TABLE 2–8. LABORATORY FINDINGS IN GALLSTONE AND ALCOHOLIC ACUTE PANCREATITIS*

	GALLSTONE PANCREATITIS (64 PATIENTS)	ALCOHOLIC PANCREATITIS (46 PATIENTS)
Serum amylase	1855 ± 213 units	807 ± 105
Serum bilirubin	2.4 ± 0.3 mg/100 ml	1.6 ± 0.3
SGOT	123 ± 17 units	78 ± 30
LDH	80 ± 12	65 ± 8
Alkaline phosphatase	73 ± 7	52 ± 6

*From Paloyan, D., and Simonowitz, D.: Diagnostic considerations in acute alcoholic and gallstone pancreatitis. Am. J. Surg. 132:330, 1976.

masked in patients with acute pancreatitis secondary to primary hyperparathyroidism, but the frequency of this phenomenon is poorly documented. Hypokalemia and hypomagnesemia are relatively infrequent complications. An elevation of serum bilirubin occurs in 20 to 30 per cent of patients with acute pancreatitis and is often accompanied by minor elevations in serum aminotransferases (transaminases) and serum alkaline phosphatase. A low level of serum albumin carries a poor prognosis. The usefulness of elevated levels of methemalbumin in the blood in identifying patients with acute hemorrhagic pancreatitis is controversial. It is not specific for pancreatitis and on rare occasions may be normal in patients with hemorrhagic pancreatitis, but it is usually normal in patients with acute edematous pancreatitis when surgical confirmation is available.[18, 68, 103, 113] Table 2–8 shows the laboratory findings in acute gallstone pancreatitis compared with those in alcoholic pancreatitis.[161]

Transient elevations in serum and urine glucose occur in one fourth to one half of patients with acute pancreatitis, but permanent hyperglycemia (diabetes mellitus) is unusual. Hyperlipidemia, including a turbid serum, occurs in about 10 per cent of patients with acute pancreatitis, but this may be due to primary hyperlipidemia or secondary to acute alcohol intoxication.

Radiologic Studies

Radiologic studies in acute pancreatitis can be helpful in confirming the diagnosis or suggesting alternative diagnoses. Dilated sentinel loops of the small intestine and the colon "cut-off sign" occur relatively infrequently in acute pancreatitis but serve to raise the question of pancreatitis for the clinician. The commonest roentgenologic finding is nonspecific ileus.[150, 157] A third of 30 consecutive patients with acute pancreatitis had no significant abnormalities on a survey film of the abdomen.[138] Air beneath the diaphragm indicates a perforated viscus. The chest roentgenogram may show a pleural effusion, more commonly on the left side, or atelectasis above the hemidiaphragm.[157] A soft tissue mass representing a pseudocyst may appear in the mediastinum or displace the stomach, intestine or ureters. Angiography demonstrates increased vascularity but has no diagnostic value.[1]

Recently the possibility of detecting enlargement of the pancreas or the development of pseudocysts by ultrasonography or computerized axial tomography (CAT scans) has become a subject of considerable interest.[45] There seems to be no doubt that both modalities can detect pseudocysts in acute pancreatitis with a frequency now reaching 15 to 30 per cent.[26, 73] There is no evidence that the more expensive and radiation-exposing CAT scan is superior. It should be noted that a pseudocyst can coexist with carcinoma of the pancreas.[58] In the problem of determining the size of the pancreas, comparisons of the two techniques have been inconclusive. Figure 2–2 shows a diagrammatic illustration of measurement of the width of the pancreatic head and body on CAT scan. Increases in size have been shown in acute pancreatitis. Figure 3–6 shows enlargement of the pancreas as demonstrated on a CAT scan in a patient with pancreatitis, and Figure 3–5 shows a pseudocyst on an ultrasonograph. Until these techniques became available the only method of detecting pancreatic enlargement in acute pancreatitis was by demonstrating displacement by the pancreas of, or its encroachment on, a barium- or air-filled duodenum or stomach. ERCP should not be performed to demonstrate pseudocysts in patients with acute pancreatitis.[190]

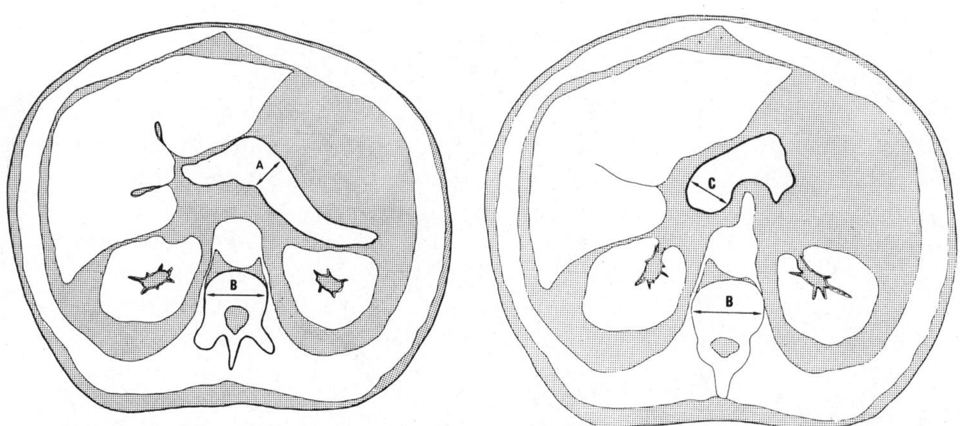

Figure 2–2. The size of the pancreas as determined by ultrasonography; diagrammatic representation. *A,* Transverse diameter of the body of the pancreas; *B,* transverse diameter of the vertebral body; *C,* transverse diameter of the head of the pancreas. (From Haaga, J. R., Alfidi, R. J., Zelch, M. G., Meany, T. F., Boller, M., Gonzalez, G., and Jelden, G. L.: Computed tomography of the pancreas. Radiology 120:590, 1976.)

DIAGNOSIS AND DIFFERENTIAL DIAGNOSIS OF ACUTE PANCREATITIS

The diagnosis of acute pancreatitis remains essentially a clinical one. The history of abdominal pain, the presence of known risk factors and the findings of the physical examination will lead to a clinical impression that may be confirmed by serum and urine amylase studies and imaging techniques such as ultrasonography and CAT scans. Although the latter may first raise the suspicion of the diagnosis, therapy must be based upon clinical evidence.

The two major pitfalls in the diagnosis of acute pancreatitis are: (1) failure to consider the diagnosis in an acutely ill patient and hence resorting to inappropriate medical or surgical treatment; and (2) failure to consider the diagnosis in a patient judged to have only a minor illness such as gastroenteritis or acute alcohol intoxication, only to have the patient present later in extremis or die elsewhere. In the presence of jaundice the differentiation between acute pancreatitis and common duct stone becomes of great importance because of the availability of curative surgery or extraction of the stone by less invasive means in the latter condition. Fortunately, ultrasonography and CAT scans promise to be of value in detecting gallstones and dilated bile ducts. The value of other laboratory tests is controversial.

Acute myocardial infarction may pose a problem in the differential diagnosis of acute pancreatitis because of nonspecific T wave and ST segment changes on the electrocardiogram.[62] Serial tracings should help. Rarely, the superior mesenteric artery syndrome may simulate acute pancreatitis, with elevation of the serum amylase.[57]

THE COURSE OF ACUTE PANCREATITIS

It is difficult to generalize about the course of acute pancreatitis. Traditionally, acute hemorrhagic pancreatitis is associated with a high mortality (30 per cent) and acute edematous pancreatitis with a low mortality (7 per cent). The distinction between the two forms is made reliably only at laparotomy or at autopsy. The blood methemalbumin determination is not specific for acute hemorrhagic pancreatitis.[18] In a recent retrospective study of acute pancreatitis in the United States, the following factors *on admission* were associated with a high mortality: age 55 years and older; a blood sugar greater than 200 mg/100 ml; a WBC greater than 16,000 per cu mm; serum LDH greater than 350; and SGOT greater than 50. During the *first 48 hours after admission* if the hematocrit fell 10 per cent, the serum calcium decreased to 8 mg/100 ml, there was an anion base deficit of greater than 4 mEq/L, an increase in the BUN greater than 5 mg/100 ml, and an arterial PO$_2$ less than 60 or estimated fluid sequestration greater than 6 liters, the prognosis worsened. In patients with at least three of these factors, the mortality was nearly 60 per cent; in the absence of these factors, only 1 among 162 patients died.[171]

In another study, patients over the age of 40 and with evidence of renal failure were more likely to have a poor prognosis.[140] Hypotension, tachycardia, fever and a palpable abdominal mass indicated more severe disease and correlated with a fatal outcome.[95] The mortality tends to be lower in reports from the United States, which include a higher percentage of patients with alcoholic pancreatitis and probably recurrent acute pancreatitis (7 per cent dying) than those from the United Kingdom (25 to 50 per cent deaths in first attacks), where until recently gallstones have been the most common etiologic factor[95] (Table 2–9).

Patients with ascites, a serum amylase level greater than 1000 units, a serum calcium of less than 9 mg/dl and serum creatinine greater than 2 mg/dl had longer periods of hospitalization.

Complications occur in a relatively high percentage of patients with acute pancreatitis — nearly 40 per cent in one large series.[129] Pseudocysts were found in 5 per cent in one series of 100 patients, along with a single pancreatic abscess.

In a prospective study, none of 100 patients with acute pancreatitis developed pancreatic insufficiency.[157] In another prospective study of 78 patients, acute renal failure developed in 5 patients, a pseudocyst in 4, a pancreatic abscess in 3 and upper gastrointestinal bleeding in 3.[93]

An important practical consideration in patients with acute pancreatitis of uncertain etiology is when to perform oral cholecystography if no gallstones are identified clearly by ultrasonography. Among 30 patients with abnormal liver tests the gallbladder was visualized in only 3, but 8 of 11 patients with normal liver tests had

TABLE 2–9. ACUTE PANCREATITIS: CAUSATIVE FACTORS

	ALCOHOL RELATED	GALLSTONES	BOTH	IDIOPATHIC	
519 pts.	31.2%	46.4%	15%	184/319	MGH, Boston
78 pts.	26%	51%	—	13%	Glasgow, Scotland
300 pts.	67%	17%	—	—	NYU, New York
FATAL CASES ONLY					
80 pts.	33%	9%		12%	Newark, N.J.
116 pts.	25%	43%		18%	Göteborg, Sweden (Schlgrenska sjukhusett)
1956–1960	5	20			
1961–1965	13	17			
1966–1970	12	13			

normal oral cholecystograms during the first 4 days of acute pancreatitis.[36] In a prospective study of 22 patients with alcoholic pancreatitis, oral cholecystograms taken after the resolution of abdominal pain but before discharge from the hospital showed normal gallbladders in 20 of the 22, although 10 required a 2-day study. The remaining patients had normal cholecystograms at 3 and 5 months after discharge.[178]

The course of traumatic pancreatitis is somewhat different. Pseudocysts may be found.[209] In one study, 5 of 10 patients also had ascites, but none of the patients were jaundiced.

Intrasplenic dissection by pancreatic pseudocysts may present as splenomegaly.[220] The problem of management of pancreatic mass lesions is related to the natural course of the disease. Among 104 patients with alcoholic pancreatitis, 19 developed an abdominal mass. In 8 the mass disappeared rapidly, and in 8 more it resolved in 3 weeks to 3 months. It will be interesting to follow the course of similar masses by ultrasonography.[41] Pseudocysts may also produce portal hypertension and variceal bleeding. If there is thrombosis of the splenic vein only, the varices may be confined to the stomach. Pancreatic abscesses occur less frequently. About 4 per cent of all patients admitted for acute pancreatitis develop abscesses.[12, 24] Signs of sepsis, fever and leukocytosis are present. The serum amylase level is of little value.[159] Multiple organisms can be cultured from the abscess in most patients. The demonstration of gas bubbles within the pancreas by roentgenograms or CAT scans is diagnostic.

Stenotic lesions of the intestine, especially the colon, may develop in patients with acute pancreatitis and simulate carcinoma.[132] Rarely an inflammatory mass includes the stenotic area.[127] Most lesions are probably ischemic in origin.[91] A patient was reported with obstruction of the second portion of the duodenum and the hepatic flexure.[7]

The acute pulmonary edema of pancreatitis appears to be due to increased capillary permeability.

TREATMENT OF ACUTE PANCREATITIS

There is no therapy that has been proved by controlled clinical trials to alter favorably the course of acute pancreatitis.[193, 197] Most such studies have been carried out in patients with moderately severe pancreatitis, and the modalities studied have included nasogastric suction,[121, 148] trypsin inhibitors (Trasylol),[65, 207] glucagon[8, 51, 143] and antibiotics.[39, 90] Meperidine (Demerol) is the analgesic of choice because of the contractile effect of morphine on the sphincter of Oddi, but if it fails to relieve the pain, morphine may still be warranted.[14] In severe acute pancreatitis, most therapists concentrate on supportive therapy, particularly administration of intravenous fluids including albumin.[53] Patients may require up to 1200 ml of serum albumin to restore the blood volume. Pancreatic abscess and septicemia are complications that must be treated vigorously with appropriate antibiotics. Most abscesses contain organisms sensitive to at least some antibiotics.[24] Nasogastric or ostomy feedings were used successfully in five of six patients with pseudocysts and five patients with sepsis.[213] Parenteral nutrition was used in 46 patients with acute pancreatitis, with 9 deaths. The mortality was higher in similar patients in the same hospital who were not given hyperalimentation, especially those who were in respiratory failure, but no controlled study has been carried out.[74] Medical treatment of respiratory failure may be lifesaving. Vigorous pulmonary toilet should be instituted for respiratory insufficiency.[94] Insulin should be used with caution since hypoglycemia may occur. However, insulin may contribute to the relief of pain when given intravenously.[196] No medical treatment has been shown to shorten the period of hospitalization for patients with alcoholic pancreatitis.[197]

Peritoneal lavage for acute pancreatitis has been evaluated in dogs and proposed for use in man but no controlled trials have been reported.[180] Once pancreatic pseudocysts have demonstrated chronicity and a thick wall, they should probably be drained surgically, into either the stomach or the intestine if possible.[60] An abscess must be drained under the cover of antibiotics (*Escherichia coli* is the most common organism). A combination of penicillin and a broad-spectrum antibiotic has been most useful.[194] The role of surgery of the pancreas in acute pancreatitis is controversial, but when a surgically curable disease cannot be ruled out in the diagnosis, exploration may still be indicated.[15, 34]

EPIDEMIOLOGY OF ACUTE PANCREATITIS

Few studies of the epidemiology of acute pancreatitis have been reported. A 30-year study in Rochester, Minnesota, yielded 321 patients with pancreatitis. Cases of acute pancreatitis outnumbered those of chronic pancreatitis 3 to 1. Biliary tract disease was present in 37 per cent and alcohol abuse in 19 per cent.[158] There was no difference between the sexes. The study covered the period 1940 to 1969. It would be interesting to repeat it now to see if the changes in life style of the 1970's have altered the pattern of results.

The death rates from acute pancreatitis vary considerably in different countries and according to different etiologic forms of the disease. The mortality varied from 6 to 13 per cent in seven reports.[93, 95, 106, 153, 157, 171, 197] The highest mortality was in a group of patients with no recognized etiologic factors and lowest in patients with alcoholic pancreatitis.[95, 197]

The age-adjusted death rate from acute pancreatitis in the United States has been stated to be similar to that from acute appendicitis.[137]

The incidence of alcoholic pancreatitis compared to that of gallstone pancreatitis has been found to be increasing in some institutions but not others. In general, in large inner-city hospitals, acute pancreatitis was related to alcohol abuse in 50 to 70 per cent of patients, whereas in hospitals with largely middle-class patients, biliary tract disease was thought to be a factor in 45 to 50 per cent (see Table 2–9). In Sweden the importance of alcohol in acute pancreatitis surpassed that of biliary tract disease in the 1960's.[195] Acute pancreatitis was severe in patients with alcohol abuse and carried a mortality of 11 per cent.[100] There was no difference in the amount of alcohol consumed or the duration of alcohol abuse between black veterans with acute pancreatitis and those with chronic pancreatitis in Baltimore.[52]

In Marseilles, the average patient with acute pancreatitis was 57 years old at the onset of acute pancreatitis, compared with 38 years of age for those with chronic calcifying pancreatitis.[183] Patients with acute pancreatitis consumed an average of 93 gm of alcohol a day, compared with 57 gm a day for controls matched for age, sex, race and profession.[182]

As might be expected, it was found that biliary tract disease is more common in women (57 per cent) as a factor in acute pancreatitis than in men.[106]

PATHOPHYSIOLOGY OF ACUTE PANCREATITIS

There are four major components to current concepts of the pathophysiology of acute pancreatitis: (1) obstruction of the major pancreatic duct, ampulla of Vater, or duodenum; (2) a change in permeability of the pancreatic ducts, permitting injurious substances to penetrate into the pancreatic parenchyma; (3) activation of precursors of proteolytic enzymes; and (4) escape of enzymes into the periductal and periacinar tissues. The third component listed may be the final common pathway to pancreatitis.[135] Clinical observations suggest that obstruction is a factor in pancreatic disease. Obstruction of the duodenal loop (Pfeffer loop) in the dog regularly results in pancreatitis. The permeability of the ducts can be increased by the injection of bile, conjugated bile acids, lysolecithin and bacteria. In response to injection into the pancreatic duct under pressure, ferritin particles can be traced into the intracellular and periacinar cell spaces and eventually into the blood and lymphatics.

There have been anecdotal reports of the appearance of active chymotrypsin in pancreatic juice from the pancreatic duct, and in some instances, this occurred coincidentally with the development of pain and acute pancreatitis.[10, 11] Others have reported the activation of trypsinogen and proelastase.[66] No convincing demonstrations have been made of active proteolytic enzymes in the tissues of patients with acute pancreatitis. Present thinking does not assign a significant role to the enzymes in the blood in producing tissue destruction in pancreatitis.

No difference in the histopathology of acute pancreatitis has been noted between the different etiologic forms of the disease.[21] The injection of oleic acid or olive oil into the pancreatic duct of rats produced fat necrosis, but triolein and paraffin oil did not. This suggests that fatty acids released by the action of lipase on neutral fat may be partly responsible for fat necrosis in pancreatitis.[185] In another experimental study in dogs, both pancreatic lipase and colipase were found to be necessary to produce fat necrosis after intraperitoneal injection.[117] Indirect evidence in patients with acute pancreatitis suggested a rise in serum tryptic activity.[6] More recently this has been confirmed by radioimmunoassay.[202] Abnormalities in the kallikreinogen-kallikrein enzyme system have been reported in some patients with acute pancreatitis in a preliminary report. There is some evidence that the trypsin-binding capacity of the blood is reduced in acute pancreatitis. It is not known what changes might occur in trypsin inhibitor content in pancreatic juice. The concentration of trypsin in pure pancreatic juice obtained by ERCP was normal in patients with acute pancreatitis, but the protein concentrations were high, and free chymotrypsin activity was present.[174]

Derangements in gastrointestinal hormones in acute pancreatitis have been identified. Basal levels of plasma glucagon were reported to be elevated in acute pancreatitis, but after intravenous injection of alanine, the levels fell instead of rising, as they normally do.[47] In another study, fasting plasma glucagon levels were normal in mild pancreatitis but depressed in acute hemorrhagic pancreatitis.[43, 109] Plasma insulin levels were elevated in the fasting state and after intravenous injection of alanine in acute pancreatitis.[47] Some patients with acute pancreatitis associated with biliary tract disease have higher volumes of duodenal content after stimulation with secretin than do normal subjects. This could represent a hypersecretory phase of the exocrine pancreas in patients with minimal pathologic changes.[48, 49]

The different etiologic factors in acute pancreatitis may be associated with differences in pathophysiology.[206] In the patients with gallstones, peroperative cholangiograms showed reflux of contrast medium into the pancreatic duct in 67 per cent of subjects, compared to 18 per cent of controls.[104] A common channel formed by the bile and pancreatic ducts was found in 30 of 38 patients who passed gallstones in the feces within 8 days after the onset of pancreatitis.[104] Alcohol given into the stomach or intravenously reduced the concentration and output of bicarbonate, lipase and chymotrypsin in duodenal content after stimulation with secretin and CCK in animals.[141]

The relation of calcium to acute pancreatitis remains unclear. In severe pancreatitis there is a fall in the total and ionized serum calcium concentrations. The classic explanation for this has been the formation of calcium soaps, with the fatty acids released by pancreatic lipase acting on triglycerides. An alternative theory proposes that calcium is taken up by bone in response to the release of unknown hormones.[223] The level of calcitonin in acute pancreatitis is controversial.[69, 223] One group of investigators found an inappropriately low level of parathyroid hormone for the concentration of serum calcium in acute pancreatitis, while another suggested that magnesium contributed to the hypocalcemia.[144, 176] It must be concluded that the explanation for the hypocalcemia is still unknown.

We have some understanding of the pathophysiology of the complications of acute pancreatitis. The transient hypertension seen in some patients with severe pancreatitis may be due to the release of vasoactive substances. The hypotension and shock are related to hypovolemia due to loss of large amounts of protein-rich fluid into the peripancreatic tissues and body cavities. It is possible that humoral factors such as bradykinin contribute to the development of shock by producing vasodilation, but this has not been documented. Pancreatic ascites is due to a leak from a pancreatic duct. Acute respiratory distress associated with diffuse pulmonary infiltrates, dyspnea, shock and arterial hypoxemia occurs in the absence of bacterial infection. It is possible that phospholipase may digest pulmonary surfactant. The basic defect appears to be a leaky pulmonary alveolar capillary membrane.

Cholestasis with marginal duct proliferation and acute portal tract inflammation occurred in 18 of 26 patients who died of acute hemorrhagic pancreatitis.[21] Extrahepatic biliary obstruction may result from inflammation around the common duct in its intrapancreatic course before it enters the duodenum.

ANIMAL MODELS OF ACUTE PANCREATITIS

Acute pancreatitis can be produced in animals by a variety of procedures, but their relevance to the disease in man is difficult to assess.[184] The injection of bile, pancreatic juice or its active proteolytic enzymes or enterokinase into the pancreatic duct will produce acute pancreatitis.[85] Most experiments have been done in dogs. The pressure during injection must be controlled.[54] Large molecules such as ferritin can be detected in the pancreatic periacinar cell space after injection into the pancreatic duct at "physiological" pressures.[22]

Injections of elastase and phospholipase produced histopathologic lesions most similar to those seen in man.[40] During bile-induced pancreatitis in dogs, active trypsin, chymotrypsin and elastase appeared in the pancreatic exudate.[155] Injection of taurocholate or trypsin into the pancreatic duct of rats failed to increase lysolecithin activity of plasma or pancreatic tissue.[163]

A role for mucosal damage to the intestine in canine pancreatitis, in addition to increased intraductal pressure, is suggested by observations in dogs with closed duodenal loop obstruction.[179] Immunoreactive trypsinogen appears in the ascitic fluid along with amylase faster than in serum.[156]

The fact that germ-free dogs have a lower mortality after bile-induced pancreatitis than normal animals suggests a role for secondary bacterial infection.[149] Infected bile, acetylsalicylic acid at pH 2.1 and alcohol all increased the efflux of bicarbonate and the influx of chloride in perfused duct systems of anesthetized dogs, indicating injury to the duct mucosal barrier.[172] There is evidence that in rats, prolonged administration of alcohol results in a bile that is more injurious to the pancreas after retrograde injection into the pancreatic duct than bile from nonalcoholic rats.[96]

The administration of steroids to rats for long periods of time produced lesions resembling chronic but not acute pancreatitis.[25] The basal volume and bicarbonate and protein concentrations and outputs increased. Bile-induced pancreatitis in dogs resulted in increased blood flow to the pancreas if edematous pancreatitis was produced but marked reduction in blood flow in hemorrhagic pancreatitis. Dextran prevented these changes.[75]

The effectiveness of therapy in experimental pancreatitis has been investigated. Cytostatics and cycloheximide reduced ascites and the concentration of enzymes in ascitic fluid in rats after bile-induced pancreatitis.[111] Trasylol given prior to experimental pancreatitis suppressed damage. Somatostatin reduced the serum amylase and lipase activity in experimental pancreatitis but did not reduce the mortality.[115] Indomethacin, on the other hand, reduced the mortality but had no effect on enzymes or tissue damage. It was suggested that the drug might act by inhibiting prostaglandin synthesis.[116] Pancreatitis in pigs induced by injecting sodium taurocholate and trypsin into the pancreatic duct followed by a secretin infusion can be ameliorated by intravenous lidocaine (Xylocaine).[186]

ETIOLOGY OF ACUTE PANCREATITIS

The only causes of acute pancreatitis that are well understood are ischemia and trauma. Cholesterol embolization of the pancreas at autopsy was reported in 23 patients.[169] In only one was pancreatitis suspected clinically. That patient had a serum amylase of 1000 units per 100 ml. The emboli most commonly originated in the aorta. Pancreatitis as a result of abdominal trauma is being recognized more frequently. Nonpenetrating wounds, particularly from the steering wheel in auto accidents, result in direct injury to the pancreas with rupture of the ducts. In one study, pseudocysts resulted in 10 per cent, pancreatic abscess in 8 per cent and pancreatic fistulas in 31 per cent. Most fistulas close within less than 4 weeks.[153]

Postoperative pancreatitis is most likely the result of trauma to the pancreas during surgery, particularly that directed toward the stomach, duodenum and biliary tract.[167] Many patients have elevations of serum amylase after laparotomy without developing clinical signs of pancreatitis.

A variety of viral infections have been implicated in acute pancreatitis, primarily on the basis of serum agglutinins and experimental pancreatitis following the inoculation of animals with the virus. Enteroviruses, Coxsackie virus and mumps virus have been involved most often.[31, 92] Enteroviruses can be isolated from the feces or urine in some patients but are not necessarily of clinical importance.[13] Acute pancreatitis has been reported in the course of infectious mononucleosis in an 18-year old youth.[226] The factors determining localization of the virus in the pancreas and its mechanism of action on pancreatic cells are unknown.

Hyperparathyroidism is associated with acute pancreatitis in a small number of patients. It is assumed that this is in some unknown way related to chronic hypercalcemia.[168]

The association of acute pancreatitis and hyperlipidemia was first noted in the relation of recurrent episodes of abdominal pain to hyperlipidemia. At surgery some of these patients had documented pancreatitis.[30] It became evident that the serum amylase was an unreliable diagnostic aid, since amylase activity was inhibited by hyperlipidemia in some patients.[219] Subsequently it was recognized that hyperlipidemia in acute pancreatitis could be secondary to acute alcohol abuse.[78] In patients with hereditary hyperlipidemias, usually Type I, IV or V, the lipid abnormality persists after the pancreatitis has subsided. In one well documented patient with Type I hyperlipidemia, the basic defect was a lack of apolipoprotein CII.[28] The level of blood lipids (greater than 100 mg/100 ml of serum triglycerides) may be of primary importance in pancreatitis associated with hyperlipidemias, regardless of the mechanism.[42, 56, 200] There is anecdotal evidence that control of the hyperlipidemia may prevent subsequent attacks.

Drug-induced pancreatitis is commonly reported, but the evidence is usually based upon temporal relationships.[32] Rechallenge has been carried out infrequently, and concomitant diseases associated with pancreatitis may be present. Nevertheless, acute pancreatitis has been reported in an impressive number of patients after administration of steroids (in some for treatment of lupus),[84] azathioprine,[84] furosemide,[29] and phenformin.[33] Azathioprine has been associated with acute pancreatitis in patients receiving the drug for the treatment of Crohn's disease.[101, 152, 160] One of these patients was rechallenged, and a recurrence of pancreatitis followed.[152] Lactic acidosis has been suggested as a directly injurious mechanism of drug-induced pancreatitis.[33] Large intravenous doses of steroids may produce marked increases in serum amylase with a return to normal in 2 to 3 days.[199] Combinations of azathioprine and steroids have been associated with pancreatitis in patients with systemic lupus erythematosus, including children.[84, 175] Acute hemorrhagic pancreatitis may occur as a terminal event in fulminant hepatitis or after renal transplantation.[83, 165] These patients have frequently been receiving both corticosteroids and immunosuppressive drugs, so that the cause of the pancreatitis is obscured. There appears to be an increased incidence of acute pancreatitis in patients with chronic renal failure with or without malignant hypertension.[16] Scorpion bites are an important cause of pancreatitis in Trinidad. The toxin increases the exocrine secretion of the pancreas in experimental animals.[17] Certain drugs act directly on pancreatic acinar cells to interfere with secretion.[191]

Mechanical obstruction of the pancreatic duct due to duodenal obstruction in Crohn's disease, or possibly in relation to mechanical pressure from perivaterian duodenal diverticula may lead to pancreatitis.[147] Acute pancreatitis has been reported in aberrant pancreatic tissue in the stomach.[77]

An association between carcinoma of the pancreas and acute pancreatitis has been noted in which clinically evident pancreatitis occurred prior to the recognition of the pancreatic carcinoma.[63] Extensive metastatic carcinoma to the pancreas with acute pancreatitis and a pseudocyst has also been reported.[151]

The possibility that acute pancreatitis might be an autoimmune disease has been examined. Antipancreatic antibodies have been demonstrated in the serum of about one third of the patients with acute pancreatitis and in 2 per cent of controls. This may be a secondary phenomenon since the antibodies usually appeared after the first week of the disease.[118] The antigen appeared to be located in the microsomes and may be organ specific.

Acute pancreatitis was associated with pregnancy, usually during the 11th to 29th weeks, in 8 among 51 women between the ages of 15 and 50 years with acute pancreatitis.[99] It recurred during the same pregnancy in three patients. Only one patient had gallstones, although six were jaundiced. The mechanism is unknown.

In a single instance acute pancreatitis was reported in a patient with acute intermittent porphyria without overt hemolysis.[110]

The most common etiologic factors in acute pancreatitis are

alcohol and gallstones. No clear-cut relationship has been determined between the amount of alcohol consumed and the risk of acute pancreatitis.[97] There is no satisfactory animal model for acute pancreatitis in man.

In gallstone pancreatitis the relationship between the attack of pancreatitis and the recovery of gallstones in the feces suggests that stones must enter the common duct to produce pancreatitis.[3, 4] Clofibrate treatment of atherosclerosis and hyperlipidemia was reported to have been associated with acute pancreatitis in three patients, all of whom had gallstones.[44]

Finally there is the entity of hereditary pancreatitis, which follows a course similar to that of alcoholic pancreatitis except that it occurs earlier in life and in persons who abstain from alcohol. Transmission is thought to be by non-sex-linked mendelian dominance with poor penetrance and incomplete recessiveness.

SCREENING MEASURES FOR ACUTE PANCREATITIS

At present, the only practical screening measure for acute pancreatitis is the determination of amylase in the blood and urine of all patients with abdominal pain of uncertain etiology. Its cost-effectiveness is unknown. Ultrasonography as the initial diagnostic study in patients with suspected pancreatitis or gallstone disease may also prove to be of value.

PREVENTION OF ACUTE PANCREATITIS

To the extent that alcoholism is preventable, the incidence of acute pancreatitis could be markedly reduced as well. The prevention of high-speed auto accidents would avoid many cases of traumatic pancreatitis. It remains to be seen whether modifications of diet will reduce the incidence of cholesterol gallstones. Avoidance of over-filling of the ducts during ERCP will prevent clinical pancreatitis as a complication of that procedure.

REFERENCES

1. Aakhus, T., Hofsli, M., and Vestad, E.: Angiography in acute pancreatitis. Acta Radiol. 8:119–128, 1969
2. Abruzzo, J. L., Homa, M., Houck, J. C., and Coffey, R. J.: Significance of the serum amylase determination. Ann. Surg. 47:921–930, 1958
3. Acosta, J. M., and Ledesma, C. L.: Gallstone migration as a cause of acute pancreatitis. New Eng. J. Med. 290:484–486, 1974
4. Acosta, J. M., Rossi, R., and Ledesma, C. L.: The usefulness of stool screening for

diagnosing cholelithiasis in acute pancreatitis. A description of the technique. Am. J. Dig. Dis. 22:168–172, 1977

5. Adams, J. T., Libertino, J. A., and Schwartz, S. I.: Significance of an elevated serum amylase. Surgery 63:877–884, 1968.

6. Adham, N. F., Dyce, B., and Haverback, B. J.: Trypsin binding α-2-macroglobulin in patients with acute pancreatitis. Gastroenterology 62:365–372, 1972

7. Agrawal, N. M., Gyr, N., McDowell, W., and Font, R. G.: Intestinal obstruction due to acute pancreatitis: Case report and review of literature. Am. J. Dig. Dis. 19:179–185, 1974

8. Alazabal, O., and Fuller, R.: Failure of glucagon in the treatment of alcoholic pancreatitis. Gastroenterology 74:489–491, 1978.

9. Albo, R., Silen, W., and Goldman, L.: A critical clinical analysis of acute pancreatitis. Arch. Surg. 86:1032–1038, 1963

10. Allan, B. J., Tournut, R., and White, T. T.: Intraductal activation of human pancreatic zymogens. New Eng. J. Med. 288:266, 1973

11. Allan, B. J., Tournut, R., and White, T. T.: Intraductal activation of pancreatic zymogens behind a carcinoma of the pancreas. Gastroenterology 65:412–418, 1973

12. Altemeier, W. A., and Alexander, J. W.: Pancreatic abscess. A study of 32 cases. Arch. Surg. 87:80–89, 1963

13. Arnesjo, B., Edén, T., Ihse, T., Nordenfeldt, E., and Ursing, B.: Enterovirus infections in acute pancreatitis. A possible etiological connection. Scand. J. Gastroenterol. 11:645–650, 1976

14. Auslander, M. O., and Janowitz, H. D.: Drug therapy of acute pancreatitis. Clin. Gastroenterol. 8:219–227, 1979

15. Babb, R. R.: The role of surgery in acute pancreatitis. Am. J. Dig. Dis. 21:672–676, 1976

16. Barcenas, C. G., Gonzalez-Molina, M., and Hull, A. R.: Association between acute pancreatitis and malignant hypertension with renal failure. Arch. Intern. Med. 138:1254–1256, 1978

17. Bartholomew, C., Murphy, J. J., McGeeney, K. F., and Fitzgerald, O.: Exocrine pancreatic response to the venom of the scorpion, Tityus trinitatis. Gut 18:623–625, 1977

18. Battersby, C., and Green, M. K.: The surgical significance of methaemalbumin-aemia, Gut 12:995–1000, 1971

19. Berk, J. E.: New dimensions in the laboratory diagnosis of pancreatic disease. Am. J. Gastroenterol. 69:417–427, 1978

20. Berk, J. E., Shimamura, J., and Fridhandler, L.: Amylase changes in disorders of the lung. Gastroenterology 74:1313–1317, 1978

21. Blenkinsopp, W. K.: The liver and pancreas in acute necrotizing pancreatitis. J. Clin. Path. 31:791–793, 1978

22. Bockman, D. E., Schiller, W. R., and Anderson, M. C.: Route of retrograde flow in the exocrine pancreas during ductal hypertension. Arch. Surg. 103:321–329, 1971

23. Bogoch, A., Roth, J. L. A., and Bockus, H. L.: Effects of morphine on serum amylase and lipase. Gastroenterology 26:697–708, 1954

24. Bolooki, H., Jaffe, B., and Gliedman, M. L.: Pancreatic abscesses and lesser omental sac collections. Surg. Gynecol. Obstet. 126:1301–1308, 1968

25. Bourcy, J., and Sarles, H.: Secretory pattern and pathological study of the pancreas of steroid-treated rats. Am. J. Dig. Dis. 23:385–480, 1978

26. Bradley, E. L., Gonzalez, A. C., and Clements, J. L.: Acute pancreatic pseudo-cysts: incidence and implications. Ann. Surg. 184:734–737, 1976

27. Bradley, E. L., and Salam, A. A.: Hyperbilirubinemia in inflammatory pancreatic disease. Natural history and management. Ann. Surg. 188:626–629, 1978

28. Breckenridge, W. C., Little, J. A., and Steiner, G.: Hypertriglyceridemia associat-ed with deficiency of apolipoproteinemia CII. New Eng. J. Med. 298:1265–1273, 1978

29. Call, T., Malarkey, W. B., and Thomas, F. B.: Acute pancreatitis secondary to furosemide with associated hyperlipidemia. Am. J. Dig Dis. 22:835–838, 1977

30. Cameron, J. L., Capuzzi, D. M., Zuidema, G. D., and Margolis, S.: Acute

pancreatitis with hyperlipemia: Incidence of lipid abnormalities in acute pancreatitis. Ann. Surg. 177:483–489, 1973

31. Capner, P., Lendrum, R., Jeffries, D. J., and Walker, G.: Viral antibody studies in pancreatic disease. Gut 16:866–870, 1975

32. Caulin, C.: Les troubles digestifs d'origine médicamenteuse. Presse Méd. 79:2230–2237, 1971

33. Chase, H. S., and Mogan, G. R.: Phenformin-associated pancreatitis. Ann. Intern. Med. 87:314–315, 1977

34. Cohen, R., Priestley, J. B., and Gross, J. B.: Abdominal surgery in the presence of acute pancreatitis. Mayo Clin. Proc. 44:309–317, 1969

35. Colman, R. W., Mason, J. W., and Sherry, S.: The kallikreinogen-kallikrein enzyme system of human plasma. Ann. Intern. Med. 71:763–773, 1969

36. Corbett, D. B., Loeb, P. M., and Peterson, W. L.: Gallbladder opacification in acute pancreatitis. Gastroenterology 74:1118, 1978

37. Corlette, M. B., Dratch, M., and Sorger K.: Amylase elevation attributable to an ovarian neoplasm. Gastroenterology 74:907–909, 1978

38. Corrodi, P., Knoblauch, M., Binswanger, U., Scholzel, E.,and Largiader, F.: Pancreatitis after renal transplantation. Gut 16:285–289, 1975

39. Craig, R. M., Dordal, E., and Myles, L.: The use of ampicillin in acute pancreatitis (letter). Ann. Intern. Med. 83:831–832, 1975

40. Creutzfeldt, W., and Schmidt, H.: Aetiology and pathogenesis of pancreatitis. Scand. J. Gastroenterol. 5:Suppl. 6, pp. 41–62, 1970

41. Czaja, A. J., Fisher, M., and Marin, G. A.: Spontaneous resolution of pancreatic masses (pseudocysts). Arch. Intern. Med. 135:558–562, 1975

42. Davidoff, F., Tishler, S., and Rosoff, C.: Marked hyperlipidemia and pancreatitis associated with oral contraceptive therapy. New Eng. J. Med. 289:552–555, 1973

43. Day, J. L., Knight, M., and Condon, J. R.: The role of pancreatic glucagon in the pathogenesis of acute pancreatitis. Clin. Sci. 43:597–603, 1972

44. DeGennes, J. L., Dairou, F., and Surbled-Dilas, B.: Démonstration du rôle de la lithiase biliaire dan le déclèchement des pancréatites aiguës survenant au cours de traitement par le clofibrate (ou analogues) des hyperlipidémies athérogènes. Ann. Méd. Interne (Paris) 129:435–439, 1978

45. deGraaff, C. S., Taylor, K. J. W., Simonds, B. D., and Rosenfield, A. J.: Gray-scale echography of the pancreas. Reevaluation of normal size. Radiology 129:157–162, 1978

46. Donaldson, L. A., McIntosh, W., and Joffe, S. N.: Amylase creatinine clearance ratio after biliary surgery. Gut 18:16–18, 1977

47. Donowitz, M., Hendler, R., Spiro, H. M., Binder, H. J., and Felig, P.: Glucagon secretion in acute and chronic pancreatitis. Ann. Intern. Med. 83:778–781, 1975

48. Dreiling, D. A., and Bordalo, O.: Secretory patterns in minimal pancreatic inflammatory pathologies. Am. J. Gastroenterol. 60:60–69, 1973

49. Dreiling, D. A., Greenstein, A. J., and Bordalo, O.: The hypersecretory states of the pancreas. Am. J. Gastroenterol. 59:505–511, 1973

50. Dreiling, D. A., Leichtling, J. J., and Janowitz, H. D.: The amylase-creatinine clearance ratio. Am. J. Gastroenterol. 61:290–296, 1974

51. Durr, H. K., Maroske, D., Zelder, O., and Bode, Ch. J.: Glucagon therapy in acute pancreatitis. Gut 19:175–179, 1978

52. Dutta, S. K., Mobraham, S., and Iber, F. L.: Associated liver disease in alcoholic pancreatitis. Am. J. Dig. Dis. 23:618–622, 1978

53. Elliott, D. W., Zollinger, R. M., Moore, R., and Ellison, E. H.: The use of human serum albumin in the management of acute pancreatitis: Experimental and clinical observations. Gastroenterology 28:563–587, 1955

54. Elmslie, R., White, T., and Magee, D.: The significance of reflux trypsin and bile in the pathogenesis of acute pancreatitis. Br. J. Surg. 53:809–815, 1966

55. Fallat, R. W., Vester, J. W., and Glueck, C. J.: Suppression of amylase activity by hypertriglyceridemia. J.A.M.A. 225:1331–1334, 1973

56. Farmer, R. G., Winkelman, E. L., Brown, H. B., and Lairs, L. A.: Hyperlipoproteinemia and pancreatitis. Am. J. Med 54:161–165, 1973

57. Feiss, J. S., Goldenberg, A. L., Plevy, D. J., and Luckman, G. S.: Superior

mesenteric artery syndrome simulating acute pancreatitis. Am. J. Gastroenterol. 66:476–479, 1976

58. Fox, N. M., Jr., Ferris, D. O., Moertel, C. G., and Waugh, J. M.: Pseudocyst coexistent with pancreatic carcinoma. Ann. Surg. 158:971–974, 1963

59. Freeman, R., and McMahon, M. J.: Acute pancreatitis and serological evidence of infection with *Mycoplasma pneumoniae*. Gut 19:367–370, 1978

60. Frey, C. F.: Pancreatic pseudocyst. Operative strategy. Ann. Surg. 188:652–662, 1978

61. Frieden, J. H.: Significance of jaundice in acute pancreatitis. Arch. Surg. 90:422–426, 1965

62. Fulton, M., and Marriott, H. J. L.: Acute pancreatitis simulating myocardial infarction in the electrocardiogram. Ann. Intern. Med. 59:730–732, 1963

63. Gambill, E. E.: Pancreatitis associated with pancreatic carcinoma: A study of 26 cases. Mayo Clin. Proc. 46:174–177, 1971

64. Gambill, E. E., and Mason, H. L.: One-hour value for urinary amylase in 96 patients with pancreatitis. Comparative diagnostic value of tests of urinary and serum amylase and serum lipase. J.A.M.A. 186:24–28, 1963

65. Gauthier, A., Gillet, M., DiCostanzo, J., Camelot, G., Maurin, P., and Sarles, H.: Etude controlée multicentrique de l'aprotinine et du glucagon dans le traitement des pancréatites aiguës. Gastroenterol. Clin. Biol. 2:777–784, 1978

66. Geokas, M. C., and Rinderknecht, H.: Free proteolytic enzymes in pancreatic juice of patients with acute pancreatitis. Am. J. Dig. Dis. 19:591–598, 1974

67. Geokas, M. C., Rinderknecht, H., Brodrick, J. W., and Largman, C.: Studies on the ascites fluid of acute pancreatitis in man. Am. J. Dig. Dis. 23:182–188, 1978

68. Geokas, M. C., Rinderknecht, H., Walberg, C. B., and Weissman, R.: Methemalbumin in the diagnosis of acute hemorrhagic pancreatitis. Ann. Intern. Med. 81:483–486, 1974.

69. Gillquist, J., Larsson, J., and Sjodahl, R.: Serum calcitonin in acute pancreatitis in man. Scand. J. Gastroenterol. 12:21–25, 1977

70. Gilmore, I. T., and Tourvas, E.: Paracetamol-induced acute pancreatitis. Br. Med. J. 1:753–754, 1977

71. Glueck, C. J., Scheel, D., Fishback, J., and Steiner, P.: Estrogen-induced pancreatitis in patients with previously covert familial type V hyperlipoproteinemia. Metabolism 21:657–666, 1972

72. Goldberg, D. M., Spooner, R. J., and Knight, A. H.: Reinterpretation of hyperamylasemia in diabetic coma. Clin. Chem. 20:673–675, 1974

73. Gonzalez, A. C., Bradley, E. L., and Clements, J. L.: Pseudocyst formation in acute pancreatitis: Ultrasonagraphic evaluation of 99 cases. Am. J. Roentgenol. 127:315–317, 1976

74. Goodgame, J. T., and Fischer, J. E.: Parenteral nutrition in treatment of acute pancreatitis: Effect on complications and mortality. Ann. Surg. 186:651–658, 1977

75. Goodhead, B.: Acute pancreatitis and pancreatic blood flow. Surg. Gynecol. Obstet. 129:331–340, 1969

76. Grant, A. G., McGlashan, D., and Hermon Taylor, J.: Study of pancreatic secretory and intracellular enzymes in pancreatic cancer tissue, other gastrointestinal cancers, normal pancreas and serum. Clin. Chim. Acta 90:75–82, 1978

77. Green, P. H. R., Barratt, P. J., Perry, J. P., Cumberland, V. H., and Middleton, W. R. J.: Acute pancreatitis occurring in gastric aberrant pancreatic tissue. Am. J. Dig. Dis. 22:734–740, 1977

78. Greenberger, N. J.: Pancreatitis and hyperlipemia. Editorial. New Eng. J. Med. 289:586–587, 1973

79. Gross, J. B., Comfort, M. W., Mathieson, D. R., and Power, M. H.: Elevated values for serum amylase and lipase following the administration of opiates. Proc. Staff Meet. Mayo Clin. 26:81–87, 1951

80. Gross, J. B., Parkin, T. W., Maher, F. T., and Power, M. H.: Serum amylase and lipase values in renal and extrarenal azotemia. Gastroenterology 39:76–82, 1960

81. Hagan, W. V., Urdaneta, L. F., and Stephenson, S. E.: Pancreatic injury. South. Med. J 71:892–894, 1978

82. Hall, E. R., Howard, J. M., Jordan, J. L., and Witt, R.: A study of serum amylase concentrations in patients with acute cholecystitis. Ann. Surg. 143:517–519, 1956
83. Ham, J. M., and Fitzpatrick, P.: Acute pancreatitis in patients with acute hepatic failure. Am. J. Dig. Dis. 18:1079–1084, 1973
84. Hamed, I., Lindeman, R. D., and Czerwinski, A. W.: Acute pancreatitis following corticosteroid and azathioprine therapy. Am. J. Med. Sci. 276:211–219, 1978
85. Hammond, J. B., and Mann, N. S.: Pancreatitis following the intraductal injection of partially purified enterokinase in dogs. Am. J. Dig. Dis. 22:182–188, 1977
86. Harada, K., Kitamura, M., and Ikenaga, T.: Isoenzyme study of postoperative transient hyperamylasemia. Am. J. Gastroenterol. 61:212–216, 1974
87. Heffernon, J. J., Smith, W. R., Berk, J. E., Fridhandler, L., Glauser, F. L., and Montgomery, K. A.: Hyperamylasemia in heroin addicts. Am. J. Gastroenterol. 66:17–22, 1976
88. Herfort, K., Sobra, J., Fric, P., and Herjrovsky, A.: Familial hyperlipoproteinemia and exocrine pancreas. Scand. J. Gastroenterol. 6:139–143, 1971
89. Howard, J. M., Trapnell, J. E., and Pairent, F. W.: Distinction between pseudocysts of the head of the pancreas and carcinoma of the pancreas. Ann. Surg. 165:293–298, 1967
90. Howes, R., Zuidema, G. D., and Cameron, J. L.: Evaluation of prophylactic antibiotics in acute pancreatitis. J. Surg. Res. 18:197–200, 1975
91. Hunt, D. R., and Mildenhall, P.: Etiology of strictures of the colon associated with pancreatitis. Am. J. Dig. Dis. 20:941–946, 1975
92. Imrie, C. W., Ferguson, J. C., and Sommerville, R. G.: Coxsackie and mumps virus infection in a prospective study of acute pancreatitis. Gut 18:53–57, 1977
93. Imrie, C. W., and Whyte, A. S.: A prospective study of acute pancreatitis. Br. J. Surg. 62:490–494, 1975
94. Interiano, B., Stuard, I. D., and Hyde, R. W.: Acute respiratory distress syndrome in pancreatitis. Ann. Intern. Med. 77:923–926, 1972
95. Jacobs, M. L., Daggett, W. M., Civetta, J. M., Vasu, A., Lawson, D. W., Warshaw, A. L., Nardi, G. L., and Bartlett, M. K.: Acute pancreatitis: Analysis of factors influencing survival. Ann. Surg. 185:43–51, 1977
96. Jalavaara, P., and Apaja, M.: Alcohol and acute pancreatitis. Scand. J. Gastroenterol. 13:703–709, 1978
97. Janowitz, H. D., and Bayer, M.: Alcohol and pancreatitis. Ann. Intern. Med. 74:444–445, 1971
98. Johnson, S. G., Ellis, C. J., and Levitt, M. D.: Mechanism of increased renal clearance of amylase-creatinine in acute pancreatitis. New Eng. J. Med. 295:1214–1217, 1976
99. Jouppila, P., Mokka, R., and Larmi, T. K. I.: Acute pancreatitis in pregnancy. Surg. Gynecol. Obstet. 139:879–882, 1974
100. Kager, L., Lindberg, S., and Agren, G.: Alcohol consumption and acute pancreatitis in men. Scand. J. Gastroenterol. 7:Suppl. 15, pp. 1–38, 1972
101. Kawanishi, H., Rudolph, E., and Bull, F. E.: Azathioprine-induced acute pancreatitis. New Eng. J. Med. 289:357, 1973
102. Keighley, M. R. B., Johnson, A. G., and Stevens, A. E.: Raised serum amylase after upper abdominal operation. Br. J. Surg. 56:424–427, 1969
103. Kelly, T. R., Klein, R. L., Porquez, J. M., and Homer, G. M.: Methemalbumin in acute pancreatitis: An experimental and clinical appraisal. Ann. Surg. 175:15–18, 1972
104. Kelly, T. R.: Gallstone pancreatitis — pathophysiology. Surgery 80:488–492, 1976
105. Keogh, J. B., McGeeney, K. F., Drury, M. I., Counihan, T. B., and O'Donnell, M. D.: Renal clearance of pancreatic and salivary amylase relative to creatinine in patients with chronic renal insufficiency. Gut 19:1125–1130, 1978
106. Kessler, E., and Mieny, C. J.: Biliary pancreatitis. S. Afr. Med. J. 49:2046–2048, 1975
107. Kessler, J. I., Miller, M., Barza, D., and Mishkin, S.: Hyperlipemia in acute pancreatitis. Am. J. Med. 42:968–976, 1967
108. Knight, A. H., Williams, D. N., Ellis, G., and Goldberg, D. M.: Significance of hyperamylasemia and abdominal pain in diabetic ketoacidosis. Br. Med. J. 3:128–131, 1973

109. Knight, M. J., Condon, J. R., and Day, J. L.: Possible role of glucagon in pathogenesis of acute pancreatitis. Lancet 1:1097–1099, 1972
110. Kobza, K., Gyr, R., Neuhaus, K., and Gudat, F.: Acute intermittent porphyria with relapsing acute pancreatitis and unconjugated hyperbilirubinemia without overt hemolysis. Gastroenterology 71:494–496, 1976
111. Korbava, L., Kohout, J., Malis, F., Balas, C., Cizkova, J., Marek, J., and Eihak, A.: Inhibitory effect of various cytostatics and cycloheximide on acute experimental pancreatitis in rats. Gut 18:913–918, 1977
112. Kune, G. A., Cole, R., and Bell, S.: Observations on the relief of pancreatic pain. Med. J. Aust. 2:789–790, 1975
113. Lankisch, P. G., Koop, H., Otto, J., and Oberdieck, U.: Evaluation of methaemalbumin in acute pancreatitis. Scand. J. Gastroenterol. 13:975–978, 1978
114. Lankisch, P. G., Koop, H., Otto, J., Oberdieck, U., Winckler, K., and Wolfram, D. I.: Specificity of increased amylase to creatinine clearance ratio in acute pancreatitis. Digestion 16:160–164, 1977
115. Lankisch, P. G., Koop, H., Winckler, K., Falsch, U. R., and Creutzfeldt, W.: Somatostatin therapy in acute experimental pancreatitis. Gut 18:713–716, 1977
116. Lankisch, P. G., Koop, H., Winckler, K., Kunze, H., and Vogt, W.: Indomethicin treatment of acute experimental pancreatitis in the rat. Scand. J. Gastroenterol. 13:629–633, 1978
117. Lee, P. C., Nakashima, U., Appert, H. E., and Howard, J. M.:Lipase and colipase in canine pancreatic juice as etiologic factors in fat necrosis. Surg. Gynecol. Obstet. 148:39–44, 1979
118. Lendrum, R., and Walker, G.: Serum antibodies in human pancreatic disease. Gut 16:365–371, 1975
119. Lesser, P. B., and Warshaw, A. L.: Differentiation of pancreatitis from common bile duct obstruction with hyperamylasemia. Gastroenterology 68:636–641, 1975
120. Lesser, P. B., and Warshaw, A. L.: Diagnosis of pancreatitis masked by hyperlipemia. Ann. Intern. Med. 82:795–798, 1975
121. Levant, J. A., Secrist, D. M., Resin, H., Sturdevant, R. A. L., and Guth, P. H.: Nasogastric suction in the treatment of alcoholic pancreatitis: A controlled study. J.A.M.A. 229:51–52, 1974
122. Levine, R. F., Glauser, F. L., and Berk, J. E.: Enhancement of the amylase-creatinine clearance ratio in disorders other than acute pancreatitis. New Eng. J. Med. 292:329–332, 1975
123. Levitt, M. D., and Johnson, S. G.: Is the C_{AM}/C_{Cr} ratio of value for the diagnosis of pancreatitis? Gastroenterology 75:118–119, 1978
124. Levitt, M. D., Johnson, S. G., Ellis, C. J., and Engel, R. R.: Influence of amylase assay technique on renal clearance of amylase-creatinine ratio. Gastroenterology 72:1260–1263, 1977
125. Levitt, M. D., Rapoport, M., and Cooperband, S. R.: The renal clearance of amylase in renal insufficiency, acute pancreatitis and macroamylasemia. Ann. Intern. Med. 71:919–925, 1969
126. Lifton, L. J., Slickers, K. A., Pragay, D. A., and Katz, L. A.: Pancreatitis and lipase. J.A.M.A. 229:47–50, 1974
127. Lindahl, F., Vejlsted, H., and Backer, O. G.: Lesions of the colon following acute pancreatitis. Scand. J. Gastroenterol. 7:375–378, 1972
128. Long, W. B., and Grider, J. R.: Amylase isoenzyme clearances in normal subjects and in patients with acute pancreatitis. Gastroenterology 71:589–593, 1976
129. Lukash, W. M.: Complications of acute pancreatitis. Am. J. Gastroenterol. 49:120–125, 1968
130. MacGregor, I. L., and Zakim, D.: A cause of hyperamylasemia associated with chronic liver disease. Gastroenterology 72:519–523, 1977
131. Mahaffey, J. H., Brockman, L. H., Jordan, G. L., Jr., and Howard, J. M.: A study of the serum amylase concentration in patients with acute perforation of gastroduodenal ulcers. Surg. Gynecol. Obstet. 101:129–132, 1955
132. Mair, W. S. J., McMahon, M. J., and Goligher, J. C.: Stenosis of the colon in acute pancreatitis. Gut 17:692–695, 1976
133. Mangall, I. P. F., and Hague, R. V.: Pancreatitis and the pill. Postgrad. Med. J. 51:855–856, 1975

134. Marten, A., Beales, D., and Elias, E.: Mechanism and specificity of increased amylase/creatinine clearance ratio in pancreatitis. Gut 18:703–708, 1977
135. McCutcheon, A. D.: A fresh approach to the pathogenesis of pancreatitis. Gut 9:296–310, 1968
136. Meier, D., Graivier, L., Votteler, T., and Coln, D.: Blunt trauma to the pancreas in children. South. Med. J. 71:895–897, 1978
137. Mendeloff, A. I., and Dunn, J. P.: Digestive Diseases. Cambridge, Harvard University Press, 1971, pp. 105–113.
138. Miller, I. M., and Irving, M. H.: The value of the plain abdominal roentgenogram in the diagnosis of acute pancreatitis. Am. J. Surg. 123:671–673, 1972
139. Miller, S. F., Whitaker, J. R., and Snyder, R. D.: Incidence of elevated serum amylase levels and pancreatitis after upper abdominal surgery. Am. J. Surg. 125:535–537, 1973
140. Montariol, T., Cabanis, P., Lacaine, F., and Maillard, J-N.: Sensibilité et valeur prédictive des facteurs de gravité des pancréatites aiguës. Gastroenterol. Clin. Biol. 2:785–790, 1978
141. Mott, C. B., Sarles, H., Tiscornia, O., and Gullo, L.: Inhibitory action of alcohol on human exocrine pancreatic secretion. Am. J. Dig. Dis. 17:902–910, 1972
142. Morton, W. J., Tedesco, F. J., Harter, H. R., and Alpers, D. H.: Serum amylase determination and amylase to creatinine clearance ratios in patients with chronic renal insufficiency. Gastroenterology 71:594–598, 1976
143. MRC multicenter trial of glucagon and apronitin. Death from acute pancreatitis. Lancet 2:632–663, 1977
144. Muldowney, F. P., McKenna, T. J., Kyle, L. H., Freaney, R., and Swan, M.: Parathormone-like effect of magnesium replenishment in steatorrhea. New Eng. J. Med. 282:61–68, 1970
145. Mullen, G. T., Caperton, E. M., Jr., Crespin, S. R., and Williams, R. C., Jr.: Arthritis and skin lesions resembling erythema nodosum in pancreatic disease. Ann. Intern. Med. 68:75–87, 1968
146. Murray, W. R., and Mackay, C.: The amylase creatinine clearance ratio in acute pancreatitis. Br. J. Surg. 64:189–191, 1977
147. Myren, J.: Acute pancreatitis. Scand. J. Gastroenterol. 12:513–517, 1977
148. Naeye, R., Salingret, E., Clumerk, N., DeTroyer, A., and Davis, G.: Is nasogastric suction necessary in acute pancreatitis. Br. Med. J. 2:657–660, 1978
149. Nance, F. C., and Cain, J. L.: Studies of hemorrhagic pancreatitis in germ-free dogs. Gastroenterology 55:368–374, 1968
150. Neher, M., and Kummerle, F.: Gastrointestinal complications of acute pancreatitis. Dtsch. Med. Wochenschr. 103:1400–1403, 1978
151. Niccolini, D. G., Graham, J. H., and Banks, P. A.: Tumor-induced acute pancreatitis. Gastroenterology 71:142–145, 1976
152. Nogueira, M. R., and Freedman, M. A.: Acute pancreatitis as a complication of immuran therapy in regional enteritis. Gastroenterology 62:1040–1042, 1972
153. Northrup, W. F., III, and Simmons, R. L.: Pancreatic trauma: A review. Surgery 71:27–43, 1972
154. Nusinovici, V., Crubille, C., Opolon, P., Touboul, J-P., Darnis, F., and Caroli, J.: Hépatites fulminantes avec coma (revue de 137 cas). Gastroenterol. Clin. Biol. 1:861–874, 1977
155. Ohlsson, K., and Eddeland, A.: Release of proteolytic enzymes in bile-induced pancreatitis in dogs. Gastroenterology 69:668–675, 1975
156. Ohlsson, K., and Tegner, H.: Experimental pancreatitis in the dog. Demonstration of trypsin in ascitic fluid, lymph and plasma. Scand. J. Gastroenterol. 8:129–133, 1973
157. Olsen, H.: Pancreatitis: A prospective clinical evaluation of 100 cases and review of the literature. Am. J. Dig. Dis. 19:1077–1090, 1974
158. O'Sullivan, J. N., Nobrega, F. T., Morlock, C. G., Brown, A. L., Jr., and Bartholomew, L. G.: Acute and chronic pancreatitis in Rochester, Minn., 1940–1969. Gastroenterology 62:373–379, 1972
159. Owens, B. J., and Hamit, H. F.: Pancreatic abscess and pseudocyst. Arch. Surg. 112:42–52, 1977
160. Paloyan, D., Levin, B., and Simonowitz, D.: Azathioprine-associated acute pancreatitis. Am. J. Dig. Dis. 22:839–840, 1977

161. Paloyan, D., and Simonowitz, D.: Diagnostic considerations in acute alcoholic and gallstone pancreatitis. Am. J. Surg. 132:329–331, 1976
162. Pancreatic pain. Br. Med. J. 1:921, 1976
163. Papp, M., Breuer, J. H., Nemeth, E. P., Fodor, J., and Folly, G.: On the lysolecithin content of the pancreas in experimental acute pancreatitis. Gastroenterology 65:778–787, 1973
164. Parbhoo, S. P., Welch, J., and Sherlock, S.: Acute pancreatitis in patients with fulminant hepatic failure. Gut 14:428, 1973
165. Penn, J., Durst, A. L., Machado, M., Halgrimson, C. G., Booth, A. S., Jr., Putman, C. W., Gorth, C. G., and Starzl, T. E.: Acute pancreatitis and hyperamylasemia in renal homograft recipients. Arch. Surg. 105:167–172, 1972
166. Peterson, L. M., Collins, J. J., Jr., and Wilson, R. E.: Acute pancreatitis occurring after operation. Surg. Gynecol. Obstet. 127:23–28, 1968
167. Ponka, J. L., Landrum, S. E., and Chaikof, L.: Acute pancreatitis in the postoperative patient. Arch. Surg. 83:475–490, 1961
168. Potjan, K.: Zur Klinik der akuten Pankreatitis bei Hyperparathyreoidismus. Dtsch. Med. Wochenschr. 89:1259–1261, 1964
169. Probstein, J. G., Joshi, R. A., and Blumenthal, H. T.: Atheromatous embolization: An etiology of acute pancreatitis. Arch. Surg. 75:566–572, 1957
170. Raffensperger, E. C.: Elevated serum pancreatic enzyme values without primary intrinsic pancreatic disease. Ann. Intern. Med. 35:342–351, 1951
171. Ranson, J. H. C., Rifkind, K. M., and Turner, J. W.: Prognostic signs and nonoperative peritoneal lavage in acute pancreatitis. Surg. Gynecol. Obstet. 143:209–219, 1976
172. Reber, H. A., Roberts, C., and Way, L. W.: The pancreatic duct mucosal barrier. Presented before the Society for Surgery of the Alimentary Tract, Las Vegas, Nevada, May 24, 1978
173. Rehner, M., Schilling, D., Soehendra, N., and Warner, B.: Pancreatic pain: Clinical-experimental study. Z. Gastroenterol. 14:681–683, 1976
174. Renner, I. G., Rinderknecht, H., and Douglas, A. P.: Profiles of pure pancreatic secretions in patients with acute pancreatitis: The possible role of proteolytic enzymes in pathogenesis. Gastroenterology 75:1090–1098, 1978
175. Riemenschneider, T. A., Wilson, J. F., and Vernier, R. L.: Glucocorticoid-induced pancreatitis. Pediatrics 41:428–437, 1968
176. Robertson, G. M., Jr., Moore, E. W., Switz, D. M., Sizemore, G. W., and Estep, H. L.: Inadequate parathyroid response in acute pancreatitis. New Eng. J. Med. 294:512–516, 1976
177. Robinson, D. O., Alp, M. H., Kerr Grant, A., and Lawrence, J. R.: Pancreatitis and renal disease. Scand. J. Gastroenterol. 12:17–20, 1977
178. Roller, R. J., Mallory, A., Caruthers, S. B., Jr., and Schaefer, J. W.: Oral cholecystography after alcoholic pancreatitis. Gastroenterology 73:218–220, 1977
179. Rosato, E. F., Cowan, R. P., and Rosato, F. E.: Duodenal pressure as a factor in the cause of pancreatitis. Surgery 68:837–841, 1970
180. Rosato, E. F., Mullis, W. F., and Rosato, F. E.: Peritoneal lavage therapy in hemorrhagic pancreatitis. Surgery 74:106–115, 1973
181. Salt, W. B., III, and Schenker, S.: Amylase: Its clinical significance: A review of the literature. Medicine 55:269–289, 1976
182. Sarles, H.: Alcoholism and pancreatitis. Scand. J. Gastroenterol. 6:193–198, 1971
183. Sarles, H.: Chronic calcifying pancreatitis — chronic alcoholic pancreatitis. Gastroenterology 66:604–616, 1974
184. Satake, K., Reichman, J., Carballo, J., Appert, H. E., and Howard, J. M.: Plasma levels of elastase, trypsin, and their inhibitors in bile-induced pancreatitis in the dog. Ann. Surg. 179:58–62, 1974
185. Schmidt, H., and Lankisch, P. G.: Fat necrosis: A cause of pancreatic parenchymal necrosis. Digestion 17:84–91, 1978
186. Schroder, T., Kinnunen, P. K. J., and Lempinen, M.: Xylocaine treatment in experimental pancreatitis in pigs. Scand. J. Gastroenterol. 13:863–866, 1978
187. Seward, C. W.: Diagnosing pancreatitis the first day: A comparison of urinary amylase and serum enzymes in pancreatic dysfunction. South. Med. J. 63:286–289, 1970

188. Shimamura, J., Fridhandler, L., and Berk, J. E.: Does human pancreas contain salivary-type isoamylase? Gut 16:1006–1009, 1975
189. Shimamura, J., Fridhandler, L., and Berk, J. E.: Nonpancreatic-type hyperamylasemia associated with pancreatic cancer. Am. J. Dig. Dis. 21:340–345, 1976
190. Silvis, S. E., Vennes, J. A., and Rohrmann, C. A.: Endoscopic pancreatography in the evaluation of patients with suspected pancreatic pseudocysts. Am. J. Gastroenterol. 61:452–459, 1974
191. Singh, M., Black, O., and Webster P. D.: Effect of drugs on pancreatic amylase secretion *in vitro*. Gastroenterology 63:449–457, 1972
192. Skude, G., and Ihse, I.: Salivary amylase in duodenal aspirates. Scand. J. Gastroenterol. 11:17–20, 1976
193. Soergel, K. H.: Medical treatment of acute pancreatitis. What is the evidence? Gastroenterology 74:620–621, 1978
194. Steedman, R. A., Doering, R., and Carter, R.: Surgical aspects of pancreatic abscess. Surg. Gynecol. Obstet. 125:757–762, 1967
195. Storck, G., Petterson, G., and Edlund, Y.: A study of autopsies upon 116 patients with acute pancreatitis. Surg. Gynecol. Obstet. 143:241–245, 1976
196. Svensson, J-O.: Role of intravenously infused insulin in treatment of acute pancreatitis. Scand. J. Gastroenterol. 10:487–490, 1975.
197. Switz, D. M.: Acute alcoholic pancreatitis: Effect of clinical presentation and therapies on outcome at a VA hospital. Ann. Intern. Med. 78:816–817, 1973
198. Taft, P. M., Jones, A. C., Collins, G. M., and Halasz, N. A.: Acute pancreatitis following renal allotransplantation. A lethal complication. Am. J. Dig. Dis. 23:541–544, 1978
199. Takagi, H., Yasue, M., Morimoto, T., Kuroyangi, Y., and Imanaga, H.: Asymptomatic transient hyperamylasemia after a large intravenous dose of steroid hormone. Am. J. Surg. 133:322–325, 1977
200. Tasman-Jones, C., and Abraham, A.: Hyperlipemia and pancreatitis. Am. J. Dig. Dis. 18:767–772, 1973
201. Tedesco, F. J., Davila, E., and Gardner, L. B.: Effect of glucagon infusion on the renal clearance of amylase relative to creatinine. Gastroenterology 75:674–676, 1978
202. Temler, R. S., and Felber, J. P.: Radioimmunoassay of human plasma trypsin. Biochim. Biphys. Acta 445:720–728, 1976
203. Thompson, R., and Hinshaw, D. B.: Pancreatic trauma. Ann. Surg. 163:155–160, 1966
204. Tilney, N. L., Collins, J. J., and Wilson, R. D.: Hemorrhagic pancreatitis: A fatal complication of renal transplantation. New Eng. J. Med. 274:1051–1057, 1966
205. Toffler, A. H., and Spiro, H. M.: Shock or coma as the predominant manifestation of painless acute pancreatitis. Ann. Intern. Med. 57:655–659, 1962
206. Trapnell, J. E.: The pathogenesis of gallstone pancreatitis. Postgrad. Med. J. 44:497–500, 1968
207. Trapnell, J. E., Rigby, C. C., Talbot, C. H., and Duncan, E. H. L.: A controlled trial of trasylol in the treatment of acute pancreatitis. Br. J. Surg. 61:177–182, 1974
208. Traverso, L. W., Ferrari, B. T., Buckberg, G. D., and Tompkins, R. K.: Elevated postoperative renal clearance of amylase without pancreatitis after cardiopulmonary bypass. Am. J. Surg. 133:298–303, 1977
209. Tucker, P. C., and Webster, P. D.: Traumatic pseudocysts of the pancreas. A report of ten cases. Arch. Intern. Med. 129:583–586, 1972
210. Turchi, J. J., Flandreau, R. H., Forte, A. L., French, G. N., and Ludwig, G. D.: Hyperparathyroidism and pancreatitis. J.A.M.A. 180:799–804, 1962
211. Varriale, P., Bonanno, C., and Grace, W. J.: Portal hypertension secondary to pancreatic pseudocysts. Arch. Intern. Med. 112:191–198, 1963
212. Veith, F. J., Filler, R. M., and Berard, C. W.: Significance of prolonged elevation of the serum amylase. Ann. Surg. 158:20–26, 1963
213. Voitk, A., Brown, R. A., Achave, V., McArdle, A. H., Gurd, F. N., and Thompson, A. G.: Use of an elemental diet in the treatment of complicated pancreatitis. Am. J. Surg. 125:223–227, 1973
214. Waller, S. L., and Ralston, A. J.: The hourly rate of urinary amylase excretion, serum amylase and serum lipase. Gut 12:878–890, 1971

215. Wands, J. R., Salger, D. C., Boitnott, J. K., and Maddrey, W. C.: Fulminant hepatitis complicated by pancreatitis. Johns Hopkins Med. J. 133:156–160, 1973

216. Warren, W. R.: Serum amylase and lipase in mumps. Am. J. Med. Sci. 230:161–168, 1955

217. Warshaw, A. L.: The kidney and changes in amylase clearance. Gastroenterology 71:702–704, 1976

218. Warshaw, A. L., Bellini, C. A., and Lee, K-H.: Electrophoretic identification of an isoenzyme of amylase which increases in serum in liver diseases. Gastroenterology 70:572–576, 1976

219. Warshaw, A. L., Bellini, C. A., and Lesser, P. B.: Inhibition of serum and urine amylase activity in pancreatitis with hyperlipemia. Ann. Surg. 182:72–75, 1975

220. Warshaw, A. L., Chesney, T. M., Evans, G. W., and McCarthy, H. F.: Intrasplenic dissection by pancreatic pseudocysts. New Eng. J. Med. 287:72–75, 1972

221. Warshaw, A. L., and Fuller, A. F., Jr.: Specificity of increased renal clearance of amylase in diagnosis of acute pancreatitis. New Eng. J. Med. 292:325–328, 1975

222. Warshaw, A. l., and Lee, K-H.: The mechanism of increased renal clearance of amylase in acute pancreatitis. Gastroenterology 71:388–391, 1976

223. Weir, G. C., Lesser, P. B., Drop, L. J., Fischer, J. E., and Warshaw, A. L.: The hypocalcemia of acute pancreatitis. Ann. Intern. Med. 83:185–189, 1975

224. Whalen, J., Rush, B., Albano, E., and Lazaro, E.: Fatal acute pancreatitis. A clinicopathologic analysis. Am. J. Surg. 121:16–19, 1971

225. White, P. H., and Benfield, J. R.: Amylase in the management of pancreatic trauma. Arch. Surg. 105:158–163, 1972

226. Wislocki, L. C.: Acute pancreatitis in infectious mononucleosis. New Eng. J. Med. 275:322–323, 1966

227. Zollinger, R. M., Keith, L. M., Jr., and Ellison, E. H.: Pancreatitis. New Eng. J. Med. 251:497–502, 1954

CHAPTER 3

CHRONIC AND CHRONIC RELAPSING PANCREATITIS

Chronic pancreatitis and chronic relapsing pancreatitis are differentiated clinically by, in the first, a slow but progressive advance to pancreatic insufficiency requiring substitution therapy with pancreatic enzymes, and, in the second, recurrent episodes of pain with periods of relative well-being in between. The end result is the same, however — pancreatic insufficiency with marked depression of exocrine pancreatic secretion. The histopathology of the two syndromes is identical: loss of acinar cell mass, with replacement with fibrous connective tissue, and dilatation of pancreatic ducts. The amount of chronic inflammatory reaction is prominent in the early stages but may be minimal at the end stage.

HOW THE PATIENT WITH CHRONIC PANCREATITIS PRESENTS

As in the case of acute pancreatitis, abdominal pain is the most common presenting complaint of patients with chronic pancreatitis (Table 3–1). It may be almost continuous, with exacerbations after eating, or it may occur in episodes interspersed with periods of relative freedom from pain (chronic relapsing pancreatitis). Among 50 consecutive patients in a Veterans Administration Hospital, pain was found to be mild or absent in 22 patients.[183] In another series of 101 patients, 79 with alcoholic pancreatitis, 17 denied pain.[95]

The pain may vary in severity from a deep boring pain radiating from the epigastrium to the back that keeps the patient from sleeping at night to a relatively mild feeling of epigastric discomfort. Figure 3–1 shows the posture often assumed by patients with chronic

TABLE 3–1. *SYMPTOMS AND SIGNS IN CHRONIC PANCREATITIS*

	% OF PATIENTS
1. Abdominal pain	90
2. Weight loss	100
3. Jaundice	20–30
4. Steatorrhea	5–30
5. Diabetes	30–65
6. Gastrointestinal bleeding	9–15
7. Pancreatic ascites	2
8. Palpable abdominal mass (pseudocyst)	5

pancreatitis to relieve the pain. Because of abdominal pain, patients with chronic pancreatitis may be frequent visitors to emergency rooms, where they may be labeled chronic complainers, drug addicts, malingerers, chronic alcoholics or patients with functional gastrointestinal disease. The pain of chronic pancreatitis is rarely relieved by antacids. Aspirin is often the patient's first resort, followed by codeine, meperidine (Demerol) and opiates, in a quest for relief of pain. In a large series of patients coming to surgery for chronic pancreatitis,

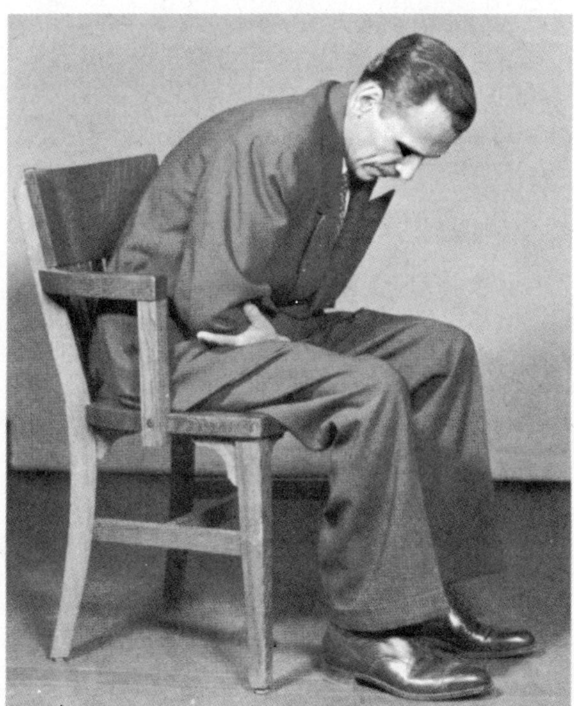

Figure 3–1.   Characteristic posture assumed by a patient with abdominal pain due to chronic pancreatitis. (From Gambill, E. E.: Pancreatitis, St. Louis, C. V. Mosby Co., 1973, p. 97.)

a third were found to be addicted to narcotics.[198] The syndrome of painless pancreatitis accounts for less than 5 per cent of all patients with chronic pancreatitis.

Almost all patients with chronic pancreatitis lose weight, but they often remain within the limits of their ideal weight, in contrast to patients with malabsorption due to mucosal disease of the small intestine such as celiac disease, even though the former have a greater degree of steatorrhea. This is true largely because the majority of patients with malabsorption due to pancreatic insufficiency have an increased appetite and consume more food.[59] Pancreatic atrophy may occur with severe protein-calorie malnutrition such as kwashiorkor, but the presenting clinical manifestations are those of malnutrition rather than the usual signs of pancreatic disease. In taking the patient's history, a daily food diary should be recorded and assessed for total calories and especially protein intake.

Jaundice occurs in patients with chronic pancreatitis, most commonly because the portion of the common bile duct enclosed within the pancreas becomes involved in the inflammatory process or encased by fibrous tissue and narrowed. The result is obstructive jaundice, although severe itching, easy bruisability and bleeding are uncommon. From 8 to 30 per cent of patients with chronic pancreatitis may at some time during the course of their disease become clinically jaundiced.

Steatorrhea (excessive fat in the stool) is described by patients as large, bulky, foul-smelling, pasty stools. The stools usually float in the toilet bowl because of their high gas content. Oil droplets may be visible in the toilet water, and their presence favors pancreatic insufficiency as opposed to other causes of steatorrhea. The patient may or may not refer to these phenomena as diarrhea.

For the patient to be able to recognize excessive fat in the stool, probably 10 to 15 gm of fat per day must be excreted. If the patient has been on a low-fat diet (less than 70 gm/day), the decreased digestive capacity may pass unnoticed. Because of the great reserve capacity of the pancreas, almost 90 per cent of the functioning pancreatic acinar cell mass must be destroyed before steatorrhea occurs. Therefore, it is a late manifestation of chronic pancreatitis. Pancreatic calcification indicates advanced chronic pancreatitis and can be used to subclassify the stage of the disease. About 60 to 70 per cent of patients with chronic calcific pancreatitis have steatorrhea, but the percentage is significantly less in those patients with noncalcific chronic pancreatitis. As pancreatic tissue is destroyed, the endocrine function of the pancreas also becomes impaired, and eventually diabetes is present in most patients. About 70 per cent of patients with calcific pancreatitis and 30 per cent of those with noncalcific pancreatitis have frank diabetes, according to the experience in South Africa. In Scandinavia, more than half the patients with chronic pancreatitis had overt diabetes, and in half of them it was insulin dependent.[110] The symptoms of diabetes are the usual ones of polyuria and polydipsia. Sometimes patients present with complications of diabetes such as pruritus vulvae, paresthesias in the feet and recurrent infections. In the past tuberculosis was a not uncommon complication.

Gastrointestinal bleeding in chronic pancreatitis is most commonly due to esophageal varices resulting from portal hypertension. It occurs in about 10 to 15 per cent of patients. The portal hypertension may be due to thrombosis of the splenic vein, in which case the varices may be confined to the stomach. Other causes of bleeding such as erosive gastritis due to aspirin ingestion should also be considered.

Palpable abdominal masses occur in patients with chronic pancreatitis but it is difficult to determine just how often. Certainly a careful search of the abdomen for a palpable mass should be made, with both the patient and examiner in as comfortable a position as possible. Masses may be the result of pseudocysts,[114] inflammatory masses (phlegmon of the pancreas) or splenomegaly. Pancreatic ascites may be the presenting sign and is most often due to rupture of a pancreatic duct in a patient with a pseudocyst.[24, 46] Pleural effusions may also be present.

Table 3–1 lists the symptoms and signs of patients with chronic pancreatitis. Fever is relatively uncommon in chronic pancreatitis unless there is a pseudocyst, cholangitis or intercurrent infection. Rarely, if the patient has been on a severely restricted food intake, one may find evidence of deficiency of the fat-soluble vitamins such as night blindness. Calcium absorption may be reduced, with resulting tetany. Thrombophlebitis, subcutaneous fat necrosis, arthritis, peripheral arterial disease and diabetic ketoacidosis all may be present as prominent features of chronic pancreatitis on rare occasions.[158]

The clinical manifestations dominating the presentation of patients with alcohol-induced pancreatitis are shown in Figure 3–2. Although the importance of alcohol in chronic pancreatitis varies considerably in different parts of the world, there is no reason to doubt that the clinical features of chronic pancreatitis are similar regardless of the etiology.[76] Figure 3–3 shows the symptoms of a large number of South Africans with alcoholic pancreatitis. The coincidence of cirrhosis with chronic pancreatitis is low but should be kept in mind. Bone necrosis is a dramatic radiologic finding but rarely produces clinical manifestations. Figure 3–2 shows the dominant presenting features of the same series of patients. Note the significant number of patients seen originally in the diabetes clinic. Hereditary pancreatitis should be considered in young patients without evidence of chronic alcoholism, and there is the rare patient with chronic calcifying pancreatitis who denies any pain (painless pancreatitis). Finally, it should be admitted that in up to a third of patients with chronic pancreatitis no identifiable etiologic basis can be found and the presenting symptoms and signs are those of pancreatic disease only.

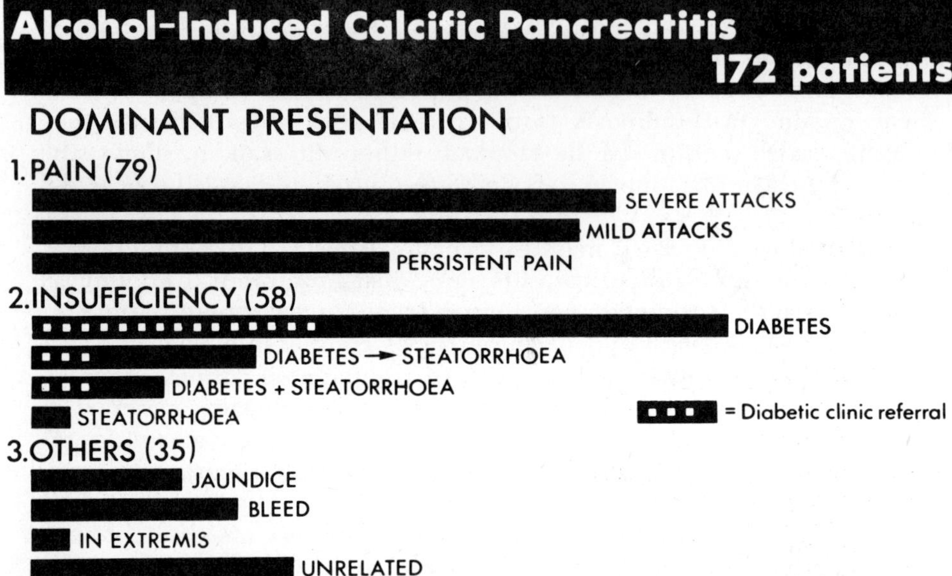

Figure 3–2. The dominant clinical presentation in 172 patients with alcohol-induced calcific pancreatitis in South Africa. (From Marks, I. N., and Bank, S.: Chronic pancreatitis, relapsing pancreatitis, calcifications of the pancreas: Clinical aspects. *In* Gastroenterology, 3rd ed., edited by H. L. Bockus. Philadelphia, W. B. Saunders Co., 1976, Vol. III, p. 1054.)

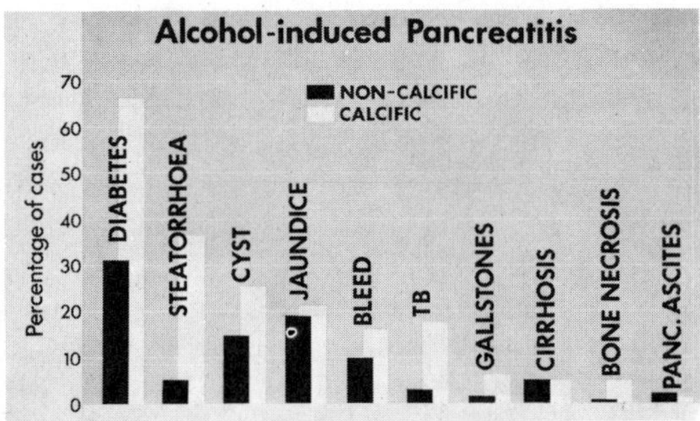

Figure 3–3. Complications and associated features in calcific and noncalcific alcohol-induced pancreatitis in South Africa. (From Marks, I. N., and Bank, S.: Chronic pancreatitis, relapsing pancreatitis, calcifications of the pancreas: Clinical aspects. *In* Gastroenterology, 3rd ed., edited by H. L. Bockus. Philadelphia, W. B. Saunders Co., 1976, Vol. III, p. 1060.)

RISK FACTORS IN THE DIAGNOSIS OF
CHRONIC PANCREATITIS

The physician's ability to diagnose chronic pancreatitis will be increased by a heightened index of suspicion. The identification of risk factors in chronic pancreatitis is a step in this direction.

Many of the same factors listed for acute pancreatitis appear again for chronic pancreatitis. In large urban centers of the United States, France and South Africa, the dominating factor in chronic pancreatitis is chronic abuse of alcohol. The pancreatitis in about 69 per cent of patients on the Cape Peninsula in South Africa is thought to be alcohol related.[118] In Marseilles the average alcohol consumption of patients with chronic pancreatitis was 179 gm of pure ethanol per day, compared to 74 gm in age-, sex-, race- and profession-matched controls.[156] This was also significantly greater than the alcohol intake of patients with acute pancreatitis (93 gm/day). In a small series of black veterans in the United States, the amount of alcohol consumed by patients with chronic pancreatitis was 1 pint of spirits a day, and the duration of alcoholism was 15 years.[54] In Marseilles the average age of patients with chronic calcific pancreatitis was 37.7 years, 13 years younger than that of those with acute pancreatitis.[157] Binge drinkers as well as steady imbibers may develop chronic pancreatitis. As in patients with chronic alcoholism in general, the physician may have to resort to questioning relatives to obtain a true account of a patient's alcohol intake.

Patients with hyperlipidemia are prone to recurrent attacks of pancreatitis, but progression to pancreatic insufficiency is unusual. Hyperparathyroidism occurs in less than 2 per cent of patients with chronic pancreatitis. Screening of 40 patients with chronic pancreatitis by means of radioimmunoassay for parathyroid hormone led to the recognition of 2 patients with hyperparathyroidism.[66]

Chronic pancreatitis can be classified into two main groups: primary, in which the disease originates within the pancreas, and secondary, in which the pancreatitis is secondary to obstruction of main ducts (Table 3–2). Pancreatic insufficiency is the end stage of chronic pancreatitis. In some patients there is little evidence of inflammation. There is extensive fibrosis, disappearance of most of the acinar tissue and large, dilated pancreatic ducts. In other patients there is replacement of the pancreatic parenchyma with fat. I have grouped these patients with pancreatic insufficiency together with patients who have chronic pancreatitis because the functional consequences of maldigestion and steatorrhea are the same, although pain is usually not a feature of the clinical presentation of patients with pancreatic insufficiency unrelated to chronic pancreatitis with inflammatory changes.

A third category of patients, those with functional pancreatic insufficiency, have a structurally normal pancreas but fail to secrete

TABLE 3–2. CLASSIFICATION OF CHRONIC PANCREATITIS AND PANCREATIC INSUFFICIENCY

A. Primary Pancreatitis or Pancreatic Insufficiency
  1. Alcohol
  2. Abdominal trauma
  3. Posterior penetrating duodenal ulcer
  4. Hereditary pancreatitis
  5. Pancreatic carcinoma and islet cell tumors by invasion
  6. Pancreatic resection
  7. Protein malnutrition (kwashiorkor)
  8. Shwachman's syndrome (pancreatic insufficiency and bone marrow dysfuntion)
  9. Cystic fibrosis
  10. α_1-Antitrypsin deficiency[64]
  11. Idiopathic chronic pancreatitis

B. Secondary Chronic Pancreatitis or Pancreatic Insufficiency—Obstruction of the Pancreatic Ducts Due to:
  1. Trauma
  2. Gastric surgery—inadvertent ligation of pancreatic duct
  3. Cancer, pancreatic
  4. Duodenal obstruction, e.g., duodenal neoplasms
  5. Stenosis of the papilla of Vater
  6. Perivaterian diverticula
  7. Round worm infestations
  8. Pancreas divisum

C. Functional Pancreatic Insufficiency
  1. Deficient release of secretagogues—celiac disease, gastric resection with Billroth II anastomosis
  2. Inadequate mixing of secretions with chyme—Billroth II anastomosis
  3. Deficient pancreatic innervation—truncal vagotomy
  4. Inactivation of enzymes—Zollinger-Ellison syndrome (gastrinoma)
  5. Enterokinase deficiency
  6. Isolated pancreatic enzyme deficiencies, e.g., lipase
  7. ? Prolonged intravenous alimentation—"atrophy of disuse"

adequately in response to meals. The defect lies in the neurohumoral factors that normally stimulate pancreatic secretion. Blunt abdominal trauma may rupture pancreatic ducts and rarely result in chronic pancreatitis, although most patients recover completely. A posterior penetrating duodenal ulcer may burrow into the pancreas and produce a localized pancreatitis. The clinical manifestation is pain, especially in the back and often not relieved by food or antacids.

A number of families have been found to have a high incidence of chronic pancreatitis among their members extending over several generations. Attacks of pain lasting 3 to 4 days begin in childhood, at around 12 years of age, and end by the age of 40.[172] The course is similar to that of nonhereditary pancreatitis. Overt diabetes appears in about 20 per cent of patients.

Patients with pancreatic carcinoma may have histologic evidence of chronic pancreatitis, often localized rather than diffusely spread throughout the pancreas. When such patients present with pancreatic insufficiency, the decreased pancreatic secretion is usually due to obstruction of ducts or replacement of the pancreatic acinar cell mass by tumor. The same is true in patients with malignant islet cell tumors.

More patients are being subjected to surgical resection of the pancreas for pancreatitis, and these patients may present with steatorrhea and pancreatic insufficiency. Since the remaining portion of the gland is often diseased, insufficiency may occur after modest resections. An attempt should be made to obtain the surgeon's operative note.

The Shwachman-Diamond syndrome (pancreatic insufficiency, bone marrow dysfunction and fatty replacement of the pancreas) and cystic fibrosis will be considered at length later (see Chapter 5), but the increasing survival of patients with cystic fibrosis only to present with pancreatic insufficiency in early adult life should be noted.[83] Patients with the Shwachman-Diamond syndrome have a better prognosis than those with cystic fibrosis. There remain about a third of patients with chronic pancreatitis or pancreatic insufficiency for whom no recognized pathogenesis can be found (idiopathic chronic pancreatitis).

In a number of patients the pancreatitis is clearly related to obstruction of the major ducts of the pancreas, leading to pancreatic insufficiency and eventually steatorrhea. Traumatic acute pancreatitis may sometimes result in strictures of the pancreatic ducts. In the process of surgical procedures on the stomach and duodenum, the major pancreatic duct may be injured or ligated, with resulting obstruction.

Obstruction in the duodenum distal to the entrance of the major pancreatic duct will lead to obstruction of flow of pancreatic secretion. The site of the obstruction may be the ampulla of Vater and the cause may be fibrosis or neoplasm. Perivaterian diverticula in the duodenum are now being seen more frequently during endoscopic retrograde pancreatography (ERCP). It is possible that these diverticula can be a significant factor in obstructing the major pancreatic duct, leading to pancreatic insufficiency.

Rarely, parasitic infestations may obstruct the pancreatic ducts, as in ascariasis, in which worms have been found in the pancreatic ducts. Schistosomiasis is associated with pancreatic insufficiency in some patients with portal hypertension.[129] A significant percentage (27 per cent) of patients with idiopathic recurrent pancreatitis have been found to have a congenital anomaly in which the two developing portions of the pancreas fail to fuse and persist, each with its own major duct. The presence of abnormal dorsal ducts and normal ventral ducts was verified by ERCP, and in one patient chronic pancreatitis confined to the dorsal duct was demonstrated at surgery. Endoscopic sphincterotomy of the affected duct could be helpful in management.[34]

There are a number of patients with pancreatic insufficiency in whom the major defect is a functional one, with no histopathologic change in the pancreas. In these instances the disease can be classified as functional pancreatic insufficiency. In celiac disease there may be deficient release of the small intestinal mucosal hormones secretin and cholecystokinin-pancreozymin (CCK-PZ) resulting from loss of hormone-secreting cells in the intestinal mucosa.[41] This will contribute an element of maldigestion to the malabsorption caused by the flat intestinal mucosa. Similarly, the gastrojejunal (Billroth II) anastomosis after a partial gastric resection excludes the duodenum and proximal jejunum from the flow of chyme, and again there may be a significant reduction in the release of secretin and CCK-PZ in response to a meal, with significant reductions in pancreatic secretion and maldigestion.

Inadequate mixing of pancreatic secretions with chyme caused by delayed arrival of enzymes from the afferent loop after a Billroth II partial gastric resection has been shown to result in maldigestion. Truncal vagotomy denervates the vagal branches to the pancreas and, on the basis of increased fat excretion in the stool and animal experiments, probably contributes to maldigestion after a meal.

Patients with gastric acid hypersecretion cause by gastrin-secreting tumors (gastrinomas, Zollinger-Ellison syndrome) may have steatorrhea due to maldigestion from reduced pancreatic enzyme activity. This can result from acid inactivation of the enzymes or reduced pancreatic secretion of bicarbonate.

There are a number of inborn metabolic defects usually recognized in infants and young children in which maldigestion results from the absence of synthesis of single enzymes.[83] Enterokinase deficiency results in failure to convert the precursors of proteolytic enzymes into active proteinases when they enter the duodenum. A congenital defect of lipase secretion has been reported.[169]

With the increased use of intravenous alimentation for long periods of time, the possibility of decreased pancreatic secretion and maldigestion when oral feedings are resumed must be considered. Intestinal mucosal atrophy has been reported to result from intravenous alimentation, and the release of pancreatic secretory hormones might be impaired. Preliminary results indicate that this does not seem to be a significant clinical problem in patients with inflammatory bowel disease once oral feedings are resumed.[98]

These examples of pancreatic insufficiency due to causes other than chronic pancreatitis may appear to be rather esoteric. When significant maldigestion due to inadequate pancreatic secretion occurs, however, one can expect favorable responses to substitution therapy with pancreatic enzymes.

LABORATORY DIAGNOSIS OF CHRONIC PANCREATITIS[3, 207]

In contrast to acute pancreatitis, the diagnosis of chronic pancreatitis can be established by a simple procedure — the demonstration of pancreatic calcification on a survey film of the abdomen. Careful follow-up studies indicate that an average period of 8 years elapses between the first attack of pancreatitis and the development of sufficient calcification to be evident on an abdominal film. The range is from months to 40 years, however. Unfortunately, pancreatic calcification represents a late stage of the disease. Pancreatic calcification must be differentiated from gallstones, kidney stones and vascular calcification. Calcifications in hereditary pancreatitis represent calculi in the large ducts.[76] The problem of diagnosis in patients who do not have calcification remains. In these patients, the diagnosis must depend upon functional evidence of pancreatic exocrine secretory insufficiency or characteristic changes in the ducts on pancreatography or biopsy. Sometimes the demonstration of a pseudocyst by ultrasonography or CAT scan will clarify the cause of obscure abdominal pain. In other patients evidence of encroachment on adjacent organs as seen with barium x-ray examinations will first suggest the diagnosis, particularly when there is encroachment on the duodenal loop or posterior wall of the stomach.[56]

Routine blood counts are rarely helpful. The white blood cell count is often unremarkable. Urinalysis will show glycosuria in about half the patients. An abnormal glucose tolerance curve can be expected in nearly two thirds of the patients.[71] Unfortunately, diabetes mellitus is so common in the general population that it has little diagnostic value alone, although in chronic pancreatitis it indicates rather extensive disease. Insulin-dependent diabetes was present in 18 of 36 patients with overt diabetes found among 59 patients with chronic pancreatitis.[110]

Amylase Determinations

Unlike the case in acute pancreatitis, the usual serum amylase determination is of little value in the diagnosis of chronic pancreatitis. The saccharogenic method of determining amylase does not distinguish between amylase of salivary origin and that of pancreatic origin. In normal subjects each accounts for about half the total serum amylase. Current research techniques do permit separation of pancreatic from salivary amylase, and there is much interest in applying them to clinical use. The level of serum pancreatic-type isoamylase was about one tenth that of control subjects in patients with chronic pancreatitis with steatorrhea.[15, 115, 175] Elevations of the salivary-type amylase levels in the serum accounted for some patients' normal total serum amylase levels.[96] Similarly, the excretion of pancreatic isoamylase in the urine may be useful.[7] The ratio of salivary to pancreatic amylase in the urine was higher than normal in most patients with calcific pancreatitis. About 90 per cent of 26 patients with chronic pancreatitis had a reversal of the normal salivary to pancreatic isoamylase ratio.[7] A group of 32 patients with chronic pancreatitis, studied by both pancreatography by ERCP and serum isoamylase determinations, could be divided into those with low values of serum pancreatic isoamylase migrating between pancreatic and salivary amylase or normal pancreatic ducts or both (10 of 13 had both) and those with an elevation of the serum pancreatic isoamylase or pancreatic duct obstruction or both (14 of 19 had both); all but one of the latter had an elevated total serum amylase. It was suggested that an elevation of more than 20 per cent of this isoamylase implied pancreatic duct obstruction.[177] An increase of two of the three pancreatic isoamylases in the serum has been found in six of seven patients with pancreatic pseudocysts. Normally the P isoamylase accounts for 80 to 90 per cent of pancreatic serum amylase, but if serum is permitted to stand, conversion to two other isoamylases occurs.[199] A venous or acinovenous pathway for lipase from the pancreas to the blood has been demonstrated during ERCP. In the presence of colipase (normally absent from serum) and during stimulation with secretin and CCK or cerulein, immunoreactive pancreatic lipase appeared in the plasma.[62] Determination of pancreatic-type isoamylase levels may improve the discrimination of the amylase-creatinine ratio in chronic pancreatitis.[15, 87] Although these results are encouraging, it is premature to predict the value of pancreatic isoamylase determinations as routine laboratory studies, particularly in the early stages of chronic pancreatitis.

The presence of a macroamylase in the serum may cause elevated serum amylase levels in the absence of amylase in the urine in patients without clinical evidence of pancreatic disease (107 of 190 patients with macroamylasemia in one study).[51]

Elevation of amylase in peritoneal fluid is a necessary criterion for the diagnosis of pancreatic ascites. The ratio of amylase in peritoneal fluid to that in plasma should be greater than 1.0. In some patients the ratio of lipase activity is higher.[173]

Attempts to measure serum amylase after injection of secretin or CCK have not proved to be of much value.[196] Indirect methods of measuring digestive function by starch, fat and albumin tolerance tests have been found to be relatively insensitive. Recently, measurement of a peptide that upon digestion is absorbed and excreted in the urine has been proposed as a test of pancreatic function. It seems rather certain that it will be less sensitive and specific than the secretin test, but when combined with a D-xylose test it may be a suitable screening test for chronic pancreatitis. Stool enzyme determinations using chymotrypsin have not proved to be sensitive enough to detect early pancreatic insufficiency in adults.[52, 126]

Trypsin Determinations

Plasma trypsin levels can now be measured by immunoassay, and in a preliminary report, patients with calcific pancreatitis and steatorrhea but not those without steatorrhea had a reduced rise in plasma trypsin after a meal.[17] This may turn out to be a more specific screening test for chronic pancreatitis than a glucose tolerance test. The latter is abnormal in the majority of patients with chronic pancreatitis, as it is in those with diabetes mellitus without pancreatitis.

Absorption Tests

Tests of absorption can be used to detect malabsorption secondary to maldigestion and to differentiate primary malabsorption from maldigestion. A quantitative 3-day stool fat study on a diet containing 70 to 100 gm of fat is the most reliable method of determining the presence of steatorrhea. The weight of the stool should be in excess of 200 gm/day.[142] Staining of the stool with Sudan III for fat droplets is reliable in detecting steatorrhea only when the patient is excreting more than 15 gm of fat per day.[50, 127] The need for doing stool fat studies in chronic pancreatitis is controversial. It may be used in following the efficacy of treatment with supplemental enzymes. The role of breath tests in the digestion and absorption of fat has still to be settled. Bile acid diarrheas in patients with ileal resections and blind loops would be expected to have abnormal cholyl-glycine breath tests.

A low serum carotene level and a normal D-xylose tolerance test may be useful findings in screening for malabsorption due to chronic pancreatitis. The D-xylose tolerance should be decreased in mucosal malabsorption in the jejunum. A small bowel biopsy to rule out primary malabsorption, e.g., celiac disease, may be a quick method of eliminating malabsorption in the differential diagnosis.

Secretin Test

The most sensitive test for the demonstration of impaired pancreatic exocrine secretion is the secretin test.[28, 36, 102, 194, 206] This procedure involves intubating both the stomach and duodenum so that acid gastric content can be excluded from the duodenum during aspiration of duodenal content. After basal collections are made for 10 or 20 minutes, an intravenous bolus of the hormone secretin is given, and collections are continued for another 80 minutes. Normally, the

TABLE 3–3. PANCREATIC FUNCTION AS EVALUATED BY ASPIRATION OF DUODENAL CONTROL AFTER 1 U/KG OF SECRETIN AS AN INTRAVENOUS BOLUS INJECTION

VOLUME	BICARBONATE CONC.	BICARBONATE OUTPUT
Normal		
	104 ± 2.4 SEM mMol/L	14.9 ± 0.8 mMol/80 min
2.0 – 4.4 ml/kg[47]	90 – 130	12.2 – 31.0
235 ± 60 SD[80]	114 ± 20 SD	28 ± 6.7
2.9 ± 0.9[28]	100 ± 20 SD	14.5 ± 7.7
	104 ± 2.4[84]	
Chronic Pancreatitis		
< 100 ml[8]	< 60	
2.8 ml/kg[18]	69	12.7
63 ± 42 SD[80]	71 ± 33	6.2 ± 6.2
3.1 ± 1.7[28]	72 ± 33	12.5 ± 4.5
	64 ± 33[84]	

volume bicarbonate concentration and bicarbonate output should rise substantially after secretin administration. Unfortunately, as this monograph is being written no preparation of secretin is approved for general use in this country by the Food and Drug Administration. It is to be hoped that the manufacturers will file a new drug application in the near future. With these limitations in mind, normal values for duodenal aspirates after administration of 1 clinical unit of Swedish secretin are given in Table 3–3.[80, 140] Comparable values in patients with chronic pancreatitis associated with alcohol abuse would be 2.8 ml, 69 mMol/L, and 13 mMol/80 min.[18] The concentration of bicarbonate has the smallest coefficient of variation, but the output of bicarbonate has been reported to be a more sensitive indicator of diminished pancreatic function.[138, 139, 185] Use of a marker to validate the efficiency of duodenal aspiration in collecting the contents of the duodenum would improve the precision of bicarbonate output measurements, but it makes the technique more complicated and has not been shown to improve its value in diagnosis.

In a recent study of 52 patients, the secretin test was abnormal in all but 4 of 27 patients with chronic pancreatitis. Most of these patients had biopsies at surgery, and while the overall correlation between impaired secretory capacity and histologic findings was good, there were many discrepancies between the severity of the inflammation and the degree of secretory failure. Undetermined at present are the advantage of using an infusion of secretin rather than a bolus[140] and of using a dose of secretin that can be considered capable of maximal stimulation of pancreatic secretion (4 C.U./kg).[47, 84, 86]

Another variation of the secretin test is to add an injection of cholecystokinin (CCK) after the secretin injection.[29, 205, 209] CCK was originally isolated from hog intestinal mucosa, and the commercial preparations still contain only about 20 per cent pure CCK. Meanwhile, the C-terminal octapeptide of CCK, which is more potent than the entire molecule, has been synthesized and is available commercially. In Europe an analogous peptide, cerulein, originally isolated from frog skin, has been synthesized and has been used as a stimulant of pancreatic secretion.[26, 79, 123, 149] The principal effect of this family of peptides is to stimulate the secretion of pancreatic enzymes. Normal values are just now being published, and it remains to be seen whether use of CCK or its analogues will improve the sensitivity of the secretin test.[26, 124, 144] Used alone, secretin is a weak stimulant of enzyme secretion, and measuring amylase secretion has not been shown to improve the value of the secretin test. Which is the best enzyme (trypsin, chymotrypsin, and so forth) or combination of enzymes to determine also has not been settled.[69] French investigators have found pancreatic lipase after CCK administration to be the most sensitive indicator of pancreatic insufficiency.[124, 160] The optimal dose of the CCK peptides is still uncertain.[144] Diminished responses to CCK in adult patients with protein-calorie malnutrition have been reported.[184]

Abnormalities in the duodenal content after secretin administration have been reported in diseases other than chronic pancreatitis. Almost half of a group of chronic alcoholics had abnormal secretin tests, and a third had steatorrhea. These abnormalities reverted to normal with an adequate diet whether or not the patients continued to abuse alcohol.[121] Some patients with cirrhosis of the liver had duodenal volumes five times those of normal controls after secretin stimulation.[8, 18, 48, 68, 73] Patients with primary biliary cirrhosis tended to have increased flow as well.[48] Others had a decreased duodenal volume and a decreased concentration of bicarbonate after secretin administration.[18, 68] Patients with hemochromatosis also had increased duodenal volumes after secretin stimulation that returned to normal after treatment with venesection.[8, 48, 137, 174] Direct collections from the pancreatic duct during ERCP indicated that both the pancreas and the liver contributed to the increased volume. It is well known that secretin is a potent stimulant of hepatic bile flow and of the biliary output of bicarbonate. Certain patients with gastrinomas (Zollinger-Ellison syndrome) have also been found to have increased volumes and bicarbonate outputs after secretin stimulation.[48] Finally, in some patients early in the course of pancreatitis, an increased secretory response to secretin has been noted. The output of trypsin, but not of lipase, was increased in gastroduodenal perfusion experiments on five patients with severe chronic renal failure who were on hemodialysis. Fasting serum CCK levels were also elevated.[136]

Decreased secretory responses to secretin also occur in diseases other than chronic pancreatitis. A decreased volume response in the presence of a nearly normal bicarbonate concentration has been considered characteristic of pancreatic carcinoma, but most students of pancreatic disease do not feel this is a sufficiently reliable differential point from chronic pancreatitis, particularly if early lesions of carcinoma and pancreatitis are to be detected.[141] Collagen vascular diseases including Sjögren's syndrome and scleroderma have been associated with reduced volumes and bicarbonate concentrations after secretin stimulation.[49] Patients with diabetes mellitus, especially those with juvenile diabetes, have low volumes, bicarbonate outputs and enzyme outputs after secretin stimulation but no clinical evidence of steatorrhea.[65] Patients who have had gastric resection with Billroth II gastrojejunal anastomosis have low volumes of duodenal secretions and low enzyme outputs after secretin administration.[204] Often it is difficult to intubate the afferent loop, but recently this had been accomplished under endoscopic guidance.[193] Patients with a gastroduodenostomy (Billroth I anastomosis) after gastric resection also have decreased volumes after secretin stimulation, but to a lesser degree.[204]

Lundh Test Meal

Probably the best alternative to the secretin test is the Lundh test meal. In this procedure, a liquid test meal is given by mouth; duodenal content is aspirated at one or more time intervals after the meal, and the concentration of enzyme (usually trypsin or chymotrypsin) is measured.[130, 208] The mean trypsin concentration in one study of healthy volunteers was 60 international units per milliliter. Patients with pancreatitis and diabetes and steatorrhea had low values in five of five cases, but low values were found in only two of seven patients with diabetes but not steatorrhea.[209] In another series, 60 per cent of the patients with proven pancreatic disease had abnormally low values.[130] Therefore, although abnormal results of the secretin test and the Lundh meal have been in agreement, in general, the meal is less sensitive in detecting abnormal results in chronic pancreatitis.[21, 81, 113, 125, 151] Similarly, it has been shown that the Lundh meal is less sensitive than ERCP in the diagnosis of chronic pancreatitis.[5] Abnormal results can be expected in some patients with celiac disease, severe juvenile diabetes and a Billroth II anastomosis after gastrectomy.[92] A preliminary report suggested that determination of isoamylases may reduce false negatives.[176]

Endoscopic Retrograde Cholangiopancreatography

Probably the next most reliable means of detecting impaired pancreatic function after the secretin test is endoscopic retrograde cholangiopancreatography (ERCP). Its findings are often sufficiently characteristic to permit a diagnosis of chronic pancreatitis. This procedure involves passing a side-viewing fiberoptic duodenoscope into the duodenum and cannulating the ampulla of Vater under direct vision. Either the pancreatic or common bile duct can be cannulated in most patients, although success is more common with the former. Then a radiopaque substance is injected, and the main ducts are visualized. Injection pressure sufficient to permit visualization of the small branches or parenchyma will lead to elevations of the serum amylase and occasionally to a clinical attack of pancreatitis. Acute pancreatitis is an absolute contraindication to ERCP. Attempts to fill a pancreatic pseudocyst also are dangerous. In chronic pancreatitis the classic findings are beading in the ducts or a "chain of lakes" sign (Fig. 3–4). Among 24 patients with chronic pancreatitis, regular main duct occlusions and variable caliber of the ducts were seen in 14 and 20 patients, respectively.[99] Normal ducts were reported in 30 per cent of patients with chronic pancreatitis.[33] An internal pancreatic fistula in patients with pancreatic ascites may be demonstrated by ERCP.[180] A comparison of ERCP and the secretin test in patients with chronic pancreatitis showed that the latter was more sensitive in detecting chronic pancreatitis. The secretin test was abnormal in 26 of 30 patients, whereas ERCP was abnormal in 21 of 30 patients.[152] ERCP can also be used to obtain pure pancreatic juice in response to secretin stimulation. The concentration of bicarbonate in pancreatic juice obtained in this way was higher than in the usual test, but this measure has not been shown to have greater diagnostic value.[134] Protein concentrations were lower, but outputs of enzymes were not significantly greater.[57] Flow rates were increased above normal in

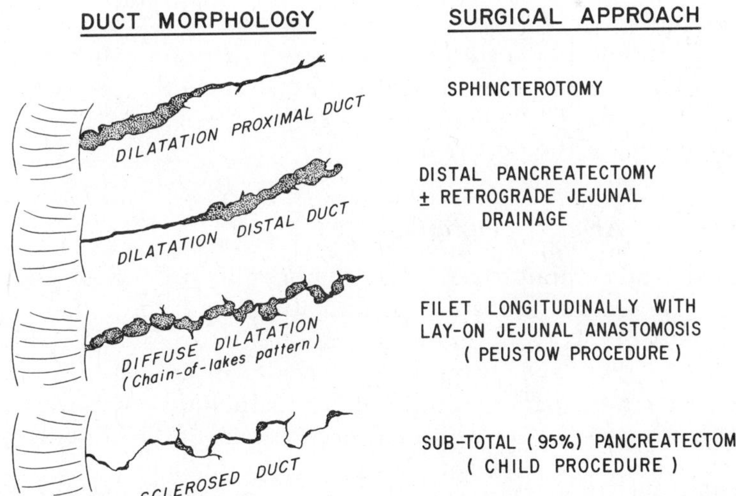

Figure 3–4. Pathologic changes in the pancreatic ducts of patients with chronic pancreatitis as demonstrated by endoscopic retrograde cholangiopancreatography (ERCP) in relation to the selection of appropriate operative procedures. (Reproduced with permission from Stone, L. B., Eaton, S. B., Jr., and Ferrucci, J. T., Jr.: Inflammatory disease of the pancreas. *In* Moseley, R. D., et al.: Current Problems in Radiology. Copyright © 1975 by Year Book Medical Publishers, Inc., Chicago.)

patients with acute relapsing pancreatitis but markedly reduced in those with chronic pancreatitis and pancreatic carcinoma.[75] In a group of 14 patients with probable early chronic pancreatitis, 12 had normal bicarbonate concentrations but low bicarbonate output (3 or 5 mMol/10 min).[39]

A preliminary report of three patients with dilated pancreatic ducts determined by ultrasonography described use of direct percutaneous injection of contrast medium into the dilated ducts.[31]

In the jaundiced patient suspected clinically of having chronic pancreatitis, transhepatic percutaneous cholangiography with a "skinny" needle may be the best diagnostic procedure for detecting obstruction of the lower end of the common bile duct and differentiating chronic pancreatitis from pancreatic carcinoma.[162, 167, 179, 200] Characteristically, the former shows a long, gradually tapering stricture.[23]

Ultrasonography

Ultrasound examination of the abdomen has emerged as an important noninvasive method for the study of patients with chronic pancreatitis.[63, 154] It is particularly useful in the identification of pseudocysts (Fig. 3–5). In one series of 17 patients with chronic pancreatitis, the ultrasound studies showed an abnormal pancreas in 14 patients who were experiencing a relapse of symptoms but in only about half when the patients were in remission.[154] Positive findings included an increased size of the pancreas, dilated pancreatic ducts and pseudocysts. In 8 per cent of patients false-positive reports were submitted. In another series of patients with chronic pancreatitis, 13 of 27 patients were identified by ultrasonography as having an abnormal pancreas.[104] It should be noted that pseudocysts can coexist with carcinoma of the pancreas.

Computerized Axial Tomography (CAT Scan)

Results of computerized axial tomography in the diagnosis of chronic pancreatitis are still accumulating, and the relative cost-effectiveness of this technique compared to ultrasonography is uncertain.[60, 61, 82, 128] However, preliminary results in 50 patients showed calcifications in the pancreas in 18 of the 50, including 9 in whom they had not been seen on conventional radiographs of the abdomen. In 7 patients diminished size of the pancreas indicated parenchymal atrophy, in 2 patients dilated pancreatic ducts were seen and in 15 patients pancreatic pseudocysts or abscesses were found. In 18 patients enlargement of the pancreas was noted (Fig. 3–6). Altogether CAT scans showed evidence of pancreatitis in 28 of the 50 patients.[61]

Other Studies

Selenomethionine scans have not been very helpful, as noted earlier.[4, 6] The value in chronic pancreatitis of secretin-CCK tests that use an injection of radioselenium to identify pancreatic proteins in duodenal content is still uncertain.[170] Scintiscanning of the pancreas with ^{75}Se-selenomethionine showed abnormalities in 15 of 18 patients, whereas the secretin-CCK test detected abnormalities in 16 of the 18.[20] However, a third of the subjects in a normal control group were also reported to have abnormal scintiscans.[20]

Selective arteriography can be of help in differentiating chronic pancreatitis from pancreatic carcinoma if it reveals encasement of

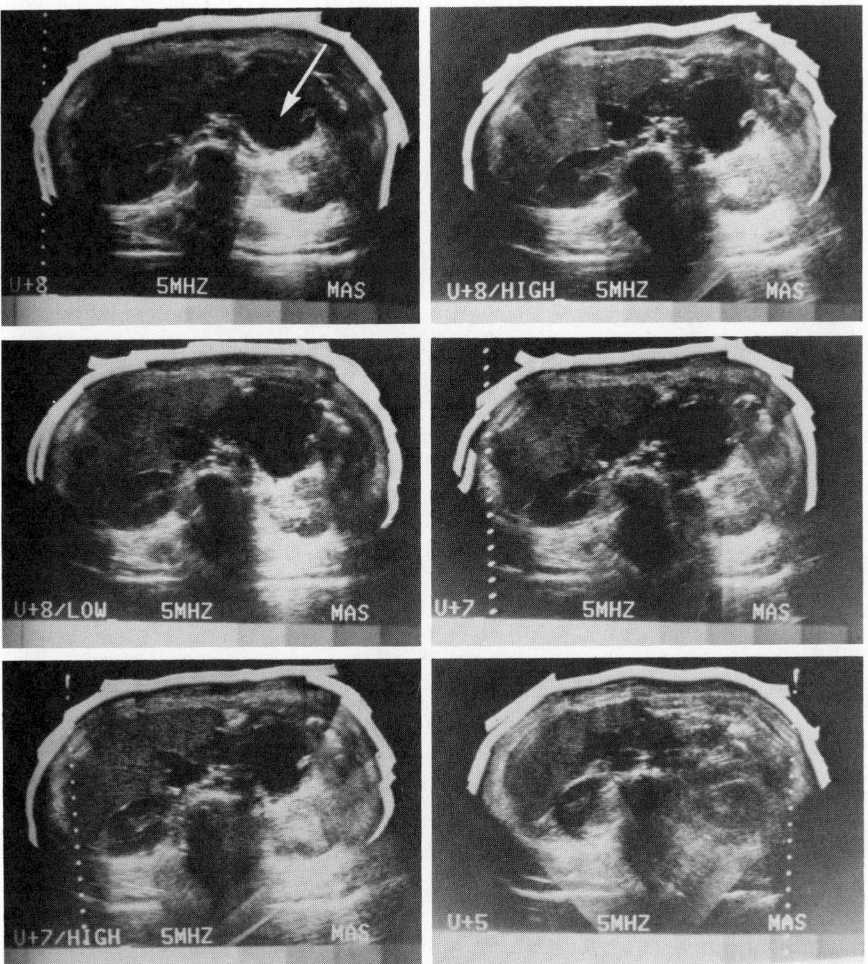

Figure 3–5. Ultrasonograph from a patient with a pancreatic pseudocyst. The arrow indicates the pseudocyst. (Courtesy of Dr. Herbert Y. Kressel, Department of Radiology, Hospital of the University of Pennsylvania.)

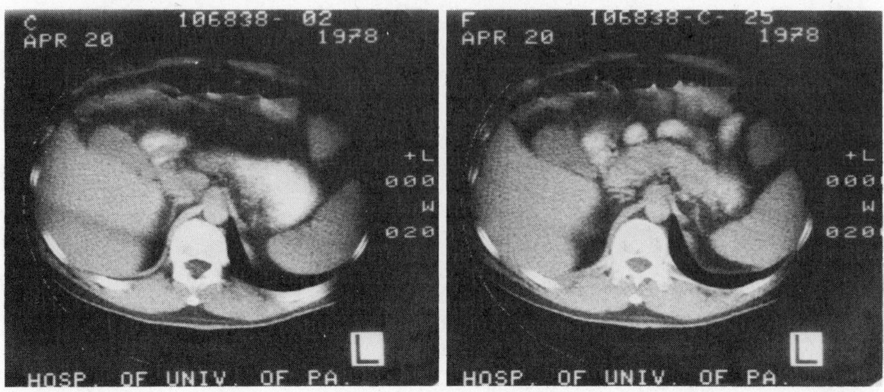

Figure 3–6. Computerized axial tomography (CAT) scan from a patient with pancreatitis. There is diffuse, irregular enlargement of the pancreas. (Courtesy of Dr. Herbert Y. Kressel, Department of Radiology, Hospital of the University of Pennsylvania.)

arteries, indicating carcinoma. It sometimes provides a dramatic demonstration of a pseudocyst, cystadenoma or cystadenocarcinoma by showing displacement of vessels. Among 42 patients with chronic pancreatitis, 31 showed increased vascularity of the gland, whereas in those with malignant tumors there was little change.[153] In cystadenomas there may be a tumor blush.

For many years pancreatic biopsy was considered dangerous because of the risk of producing a pancreatic fistula. Current methods using a small-bore needle appear to be quite safe. Biopsy can be performed during laparotomy or percutaneously under guidance by ultrasonography or CAT scan. Although at present the cytologic diagnosis of cancer is the principal diagnostic criterion, it may be possible to develop criteria for the diagnosis of chronic pancreatitis, on the basis of experience at surgery or at autopsy.

Laparotomy will doubtless continue to be employed in the diagnosis of chronic pancreatitis, but it is hoped that a tissue diagnosis achieved by needle biopsy or some other technique will replace the vagaries of the palpating hand and the unfortunate performance of a total pancreatectomy in a patient with chronic pancreatitis under the impression that a carcinoma was present.

A few attempts have been made to compare the usefulness of several laboratory procedures in the diagnosis of chronic pancreatitis.[35, 207] In patients with pain as a major complaint, ERCP seemed more valuable than CAT scans, but in those with a pancreatic mass there was no difference. CAT scans were more helpful in differentiating carcinoma from chronic pancreatitis.[35] Subsequent experience from the same unit shows that with expert interpretation ultrasonography was more accurate than the CAT scan.[34]

DIAGNOSIS AND DIFFERENTIAL DIAGNOSIS
OF CHRONIC PANCREATITIS

To be secure, the diagnosis of chronic pancreatitis requires some objective evidence of abnormalities in the pancreas. In the early stages, when pain is the principal symptom, the disease is notoriously difficult to diagnose unless objective changes, such as calcification of the pancreas, steatorrhea, or malabsorption, are present. These changes are usually late manifestations, however, and there is still no agreement on the criteria for diagnosis of the early stage of chronic pancreatitis.

The major problems in differential diagnosis are the sorting out of various causes of abdominal pain, the recognition of malabsorption of fat and protein and then the defining of a major role of deficient pancreatic exocrine secretion in the malabsorption, rather than mucosal disease of the small intestine. Table 3–4 lists the principal disorders to be considered in the differential diagnosis. The results of laboratory procedures may be necessary to exclude some of them, but here we shall be concerned only with clinical considerations.

The pain of chronic pancreatitis differs from that of uncomplicated duodenal ulcer by *not* being relieved by food or antacids. Posterior penetrating duodenal ulcer has usually been preceded by a typical history of uncomplicated ulcer. Gastric ulcers are best excluded on the basis of periodic exacerbations and complete remissions of pain in the past, when that is possible. In pancreatic carcinoma the pain is often present at night and not particularly influenced by meals. Some patients with pancreatic carcinoma may present with malabsorption and steatorrhea as the dominant features, and differentiation from chronic pancreatitis on the basis of clinical evidence may not be possible.

The pain of acute cholecystitis or biliary colic is acute or episodic or both. It is often localized to the right upper quadrant of the

*TABLE 3–4.   THE DIFFERENTIAL DIAGNOSIS OF CHRONIC
PANCREATITIS*

---

1. Peptic ulcer disease
2. Pancreatic carcinoma
3. Gallstones and cholecystitis
4. Drug addiction
5. Functional gastrointestinal disease
6. Alcoholic hepatitis
7. Cirrhosis of the liver
8. Malabsorption syndromes
9. Carcinoma of the stomach or colon
10. Diabetes mellitus

---

abdomen. Tenderness to palpation is also localized to the right upper quadrant. Gallstones occur commonly, in as many as 10 per cent of the population of age 60 years and up in the United States.

With a disease as common as gallstones, one must be prepared to find a significant number of patients who have both gallstones and pancreatitis but in whom the gallstones are an incidental finding. In general, gallstones do not cause chronic pancreatitis, but they can be a cause of recurrent pancreatitis or chronic relapsing pancreatitis.

Addiction to narcotics, alcohol abuse and chronic pancreatitis can be found in a similar group of patients. They are a difficult and discouraging group of individuals to deal with. Their histories are often unreliable, and they fail to keep their appointments and meet their obligations. Nevertheless, it is a diagnostic challenge to sort out from this group those who have pancreatitis and may respond to appropriate therapy. The most useful asset in making a correct diagnosis is a high index of suspicion.

Patients with functional gastrointestinal disease often have a long history of similar symptoms without any evidence of objective consequences, e.g., weight loss.

Patients with alcohol-related liver disease, either alcoholic hepatitis or cirrhosis, pose a particular problem because of the common factor of alcohol abuse. In a group of black veterans with chronic pancreatitis in Baltimore, more than half had clinical evidence of chronic liver disease in both retrospective and prospective studies. From 15 to 30 per cent had biopsy-proven cirrhosis. A tender, enlarged liver speaks for alcoholic hepatitis, and the presence of hepatomegaly and the stigmata of chronic liver disease (e.g., spider angiomata, palmar erythema and testicular atrophy) point to the diagnosis of cirrhosis.

The fact that patients with malabsorption syndromes have greater weight loss and poorer appetite than patients with pancreatic insufficiency has already been pointed out. Evidence of vitamin deficiencies is also more unusual in chronic pancreatitis. The pain of chronic pancreatitis is the most obvious differential feature. A history of celiac disease in childhood would be helpful. Anemia is less common in chronic pancreatitis.

Carcinoma of the stomach or colon is usually far advanced by the time it simulates chronic pancreatitis. Evidence of lymph node metastasis to supraclavicular nodes, hepatic enlargement or a perirectal shelf felt on digital examination of the rectum points to carcinoma.

Diabetes mellitus is more common in those with chronic pancreatitis than in the general population, and, as noted earlier, diabetes clinics are common sources of referrals of patients with chronic pancreatitis. The pain is usually a distinguishing characteristic, and significant steatorrhea is also usually not seen in diabetes mellitus.

Laboratory tests should be employed to (1) demonstrate that the pancreas is abnormal; (2) identify calcification of the pancreas and hence chronic pancreatitis in most instances; (3) exclude significant pancreatic disease; and (4) identify diseases as alternative diagnoses, particularly mucosal disease of the small intestine as a cause of malabsorption. At present ultrasonography is favored as an initial noninvasive, safe and relatively inexpensive procedure, but the final role of the ultrasonography vs. CAT scan is uncertain. If the result of ultrasonography is negative or uncertain, then a secretin and CCK test should be considered as a more sensitive procedure in identifying early pancreatic disease. In the jaundiced patient percutaneous transhepatic cholangiography is helpful if it is positive. ERCP may provide a tissue diagnosis in the case of ampullary lesions. Small bowel biopsy may be the most direct means of differentiating malabsorption from pancreatic insufficiency. Screening tests such as the D-xylose tolerance test to detect mucosal disease may be helpful. ERCP appears to be particularly useful in planning surgical therapy in chronic pancreatitis. Biopsy and cytologic study may be the only means of differentiating chronic pancreatitis from pancreatic carcinoma.

THE COURSE OF CHRONIC PANCREATITIS

The course of chronic pancreatitis depends upon the etiologic factors. Calcific pancreatitis in the Western World is usually related to alcohol abuse, the exceptions being primarily idiopathic and hereditary pancreatitis. If alcohol intake continues, recurrent attacks of a steady progression to pancreatic insufficiency with steatorrhea occurs. Almost half the patients may be expected to have some lessening of the pain as the disease advances, but in a quarter the pain becomes more severe.[108] As noted earlier, the distinction between recurrent acute pancreatitis and chronic relapsing pancreatitis may be difficult to make because of uncertainty about the return of the pancreas to normal between attacks. In general, patients with alcohol-related chronic pancreatitis have less evidence of pancreatic insufficiency and fewer complications. In patients with hereditary pancreatitis, thrombosis of the portal or splenic vein has been reported in 3 of 10 patients.[119] It has been estimated that 8 years, on the average, elapse between the first attack of alcoholic pancreatitis and the appearance of calcification. Jaundice developing in the course of alcoholic pancreatitis may be due to compression of the common bile duct within the pancreas. Percutaneous transhepatic cholangiography with the "skinny" needle will demonstrate the narrowed common bile duct, and ERCP may show the typical changes in the pancreatic ducts. The serum alkaline phosphatase is usually significantly elevated.

In the past death in chronic pancreatitis was usually due to intercurrent infections. Today liver failure is an increasingly common cause of death, accounting for 5 deaths in 51 patients treated surgically for chronic pancreatitis.[95] Complete abstinence from alcohol is usually followed by relief of pain and arrest of progression of the disease, but some patients continue to have pain and to show progression of pancreatic insufficiency even after they have stopped drinking.

Complications of chronic pancreatitis, such as pseudocysts, diabetes, gastrointestinal bleeding and intercurrent infections, may dominate the course of the disease. Portal or splenic vein thrombosis may lead to variceal bleeding in chronic pancreatitis of all etiologic types, including familial pancreatitis.[14] Pancreatic mass lesions may disappear spontaneously or require surgical drainage. A preliminary report suggests that percutaneous transabdominal aspiration of pancreatic pseudocysts may avoid the need for surgery in some patients (three of six).[178]

TREATMENT OF CHRONIC PANCREATITIS

The relief of pain in chronic pancreatitis is a major unsolved problem.[2] There are few data available to help the physician in choosing drugs. Traditionally, antacids and frequent small meals have been recommended on the grounds that they "rest" the pancreas. The possibility that vigorous substitution therapy with pancreatic extracts may relieve pain is under study. Among analgesics, acetaminophen (Tylenol) is preferable to aspirin. Abstinence from alcohol is much to be desired but seldom achieved. Codeine and meperidine (Demerol) taken over any substantial period of time almost invariably lead to addiction. Morphine should be avoided because of its addicting properties and because of its action in contracting the sphincter of Oddi. Eventually, either the pain seems to lessen spontaneously or the patient seeks surgical procedures for relief. If a pseudocyst is found, anastomosis of the cyst to the stomach or small intestine is often successful in relieving pain. Percutaneous aspiration of pseudocysts has been reported.[178] If no pseudocyst can be found, then ERCP should be done and the type of surgery tailored to the state of the ducts that is found. Figure 3–4 illustrates how such choices could be made. There is no evidence, however, that such a selection procedure will improve the final results. Jaundice due to narrowing of the common bile duct by the adjacent inflamed pancreas may require drainage of the biliary tract.[167, 179, 200]

The treatment of pancreatic insufficiency involves substitution therapy with pancreatic enzymes and treatment of the diabetes.[166] Commercial preparations vary in their ability to reduce steatorrhea, and there is little standardization of preparations.[72] Administration of enzymes with meals and in tablet or powder form rather than in enteric-coated capsules is desirable. Steatorrhea and azotorrhea (excessive nitrogen in the stool) can be reduced if eight tablets of pancreatic extract are taken with each meal. It has been suggested that two tablets be taken early in the meal, four in the middle of the meal and two near the end. Viokase, cotazyme and ilozyme have been shown to correct the steatorrhea under these circumstances.[43, 72]

Some patients secrete sufficient gastric hydrochloric acid and pepsin to inactivate pancreatic enzymes taken orally.[88] Antacids can help, and currently cimetidine is under study as another means of suppressing gastric acidity.[145] Bicarbonate is seldom needed. Complete correction of the steatorrhea is rarely achieved and probably is not necessary unless it proves helpful in the control of pain. About half the patients with overt diabetes and chronic pancreatitis are insulin dependent and have a reduced blood insulin level after a meal.[110] Hypoglycemic reactions are common (14 of 18 patients) and were fatal in 3 patients. Low levels of plasma glucagon may contribute to the hypoglycemia and brain damage. A trial with oral hypoglycemic agents before resorting to insulin may be prudent in patients without ketosis.

The surgical procedures used in chronic pancreatitis, apart from those directed as pseudocysts, are based upon two general principles: the relief of obstruction and the excision of diseased tissue.[44] The appropriate operation for the relief of obstruction depends upon the location of the obstruction. It is possible that sphincterotomy or sphincteroplasty owes its successes to the relief of obstruction in the main pancreatic duct, but no standards have been developed to permit selection of the patients who will respond uniformly well to this procedure. Pancreatography either by the endoscopic retrograde route or at operation can demonstrate the site of obstruction within the ducts.[100, 182] Localized obstruction within the head of the pancreas can be relieved by distal pancreaticojejunostomy. Multiple stenoses may be dealt with by a filet procedure joining the pancreas to the jejunum over a lengthy portion of the major ducts. When no localized obstruction can be demonstrated, and particularly when pain is the major symptom, excision of pancreatic parenchyma may be the only alternative. Patency of the ducts can be evaluated postoperatively by ERCP. The two principal procedures are a 75 to 95 per cent pancreatectomy, sparing a portion of parenchyma adjacent to the duodenum, and total pancreatectomy. These operations are associated with significant morbidity and mortality. After the immediate postoperative period diabetes mellitus becomes a major consideration, particularly in chronic abusers of alcohol, who are notoriously unreliable in their use of insulin.[12] It remains to be seen if the novel approach of injecting islet cells into the portal vein will ameliorate the diabetes. Operations to relieve pain by cutting the vagus or sympathetic nerves have largely been abandoned in the United States. In one large series of 530 patients, 546 surgical procedures were performed. The average age of the patients was 42 years. In 37 per cent of the patients the cause of the pancreatitis was unknown; 41 per cent had chronic alcoholism; 28

per cent had gallstones; and 10 per cent had both. Transduodenal exploration of the pancreatic ducts was done in all patients. Then a sphincteroplasty was performed in 55 patients, a pancreaticoduodenectomy (Whipple procedure) in 82 patients, distal pancreatectomy in 73 patients and total pancreatectomy in 8 patients. Satisfactory results were obtained in 72 per cent, 68 per cent, 75 per cent and 88 per cent, respectively. After transduodenal exploration, 4 patients (2.6 per cent) died of postoperative acute pancreatitis.[198]

In another series of 57 patients, 58 per cent of whom were chronic alcoholics, a longitudinal pancreaticojejunostomy was done on 21 patients, with good results in 13; a partial pancreatectomy in 11 patients, 8 of whom had good results; and a subtotal pancreatectomy in 3, 2 of whom became free of pain.[202]

French surgeons have had a wide experience with chronic pancreatitis. Of 57 patients followed for 3 years, 42 were alive and 15 dead. Pancreaticoduodenectomy (the Whipple procedure, sparing the tail of the pancreas) was done in all, with good results in 31, fair results in 6, poor results in 2 and bad results in 3. In about a third of the patients who obtained relief of pain initially, hepatic failure developed subsequently.[78]

In a study of 148 patients followed for 20 years, a distal pancreatectomy was done in 71 patients and a pancreaticoduodenectomy in 16. During the subsequent 20 years, 46 per cent of the distal pancreatectomy group died: 13 of pancreatitis and 10 of cirrhosis of the liver. Fifty-six per cent of the patients with pancreaticoduodenectomy died. Splanchnicectomy was done as an initial procedure in 18 patients and secondarily in another 13. Of the patients having distal pancreatectomy and surviving, 68 per cent had good results, 11 per cent fair and 21 per cent bad. Fourteen patients required reoperation. Six of the 8 patients still living who had pancreaticoduodenectomy had good results. Only 5 of the 16 patients who had splanchnicectomy as a primary procedure had good results, and in 9, the results were bad.[106]

The major purpose of surgery in chronic pancreatitis is to relieve pain. In one series of 113 patients with chronic pancreatitis, 43 were operated upon. Failure of the initial operative procedure led to a second operation in 13 of the patients. Of the 43 who had surgical procedures, 17 improved and 11 did not. Diabetes developed in 11 patients and diarrhea in 5.[109]

In another series of 101 patients with chronic pancreatitis, 51 were operated upon and 21 derived definite benefit from the surgery.[95] There was a definite correlation between the degree of pancreatic insufficiency and lasting relief of pain in 57 patients with chronic pancreatitis. It was suggested that better pain relief after pancreatic resection may reflect greater pancreatic insufficiency rather than the value of a particular surgical procedure.[2] Among 46 black patients with chronic pancreatitis, 28 had clinical evidence of chronic liver disease and 15 had biopsy-proven cirrhosis.[54] There was no difference in the amount of alcohol consumed (1 pint per day) or the duration of alcohol abuse (16 to 18 years) between patients with liver disease and those without it. Hepatic failure after surgical treatment of chronic pancreatitis may be related to coincident cirrhosis.

EPIDEMIOLOGY OF CHRONIC PANCREATITIS

The epidemiology of chronic pancreatitis is not well known. In Rochester, Minnesota, between 1940 and 1969 there was only one patient with chronic pancreatitis for every three with acute pancreatitis.[135] The average age of patients with chronic calcifying pancreatitis was 13 years younger than that of those with acute pancreatitis.[157] The mortality rate from chronic pancreatitis is unknown, but there is some evidence that surgical operations for intractable pain are not inconsiderable factors.[143]

There is no dose-related alcohol factor that distinguishes acute from chronic pancreatitis. Cirrhosis may be found in as many as a third of patients with chronic pancreatitis in a Veterans Administration hospital population.[54]

PATHOPHYSIOLOGY OF CHRONIC PANCREATITIS

The pathophysiology of chronic pancreatitis is characterized by destruction of acinar tissue and replacement with fibrous tissue, together with a dilatation of the ducts.[90, 161] Eventually the islets of Langerhans are also reduced in number. The process is a patchy one with a lobular distribution. Protein plugs in the ducts and perilobular and intralobular fibrosis are prominent factors. The weight of the pancreas decreases. Ducts of all sizes are involved.[132, 157] One group of 27 patients with chronic pancreatitis has been studied by secretin tests and ERCP. In 26 of the patients biopsies of the pancreas were available. The secretin response was abnormal in 23 patients: 21 had low bicarbonate outputs and 2 had abnormal volumes. Nineteen had abnormal pancreatograms, including beading of the ducts in four and obstruction of the ducts in three.[203] In another series of 139 patients, including 89 with abnormal secretin-CCK tests, there was no correlation between the diameter of the main pancreatic duct and the results of the secretory tests.[131] These functional changes reflect both a reduction of the secretory mass of the pancreas and obstruction within its ducts.

The correlation between changes in pancreatic exocrine secretion and the course of chronic pancreatitis indicates that extensive disease must be present before significant decreases in the secretion of bicarbonate or enzyme occur. With direct cannulation of the pancreatic duct by ERCP, there was no difference in bicarbonate secretion between normal subjects and patients suspected of having early chronic pancreatitis.[39] Patients with pancreatic insufficiency had the anticipated reduction in bicarbonate output after administration of 70 units of secretin (1.8 mMol/10 min vs. 5 mMol in normal persons).[39] Correlation of duodenal bicarbonate output with fecal fat excretion showed that the former had to be reduced by about 90 per cent before steatorrhea was evident.[27]

In patients with chronic alcoholic pancreatitis, juice obtained by direct cannulation of the pancreatic duct after secretin-CCK stimulation showed a three-fold increase in the ratio of trypsin to trypsin inhibitor that was due to an increase in the concentration of trypsin.[148] The concentration of total protein and output increased in alcoholic pancreatitis in man, while bicarbonate and water outputs fell.[155]

A relatively large reserve capacity of the pancreas for enzyme secretion has also been found. Among 17 patients with chronic pancreatitis the duodenal trypsin output fell to 10 per cent of normal before malabsorption was evident.[42] Duodenal lipase output in response to intestinal perfusion of amino acids or intravenous injection of CCK fell to 15 per cent of normal before steatorrhea occurred[41] (Fig. 3–7).

Very low levels of colipase may be found in some patients with pancreatic insufficiency and steatorrhea and may contribute to the steatorrhea, particularly when the lipase activity is also much reduced.[67] Confirmation of these observations comes from studies of fat absorption in patients after surgical resection of the pancreas. Among seven patients who had had resection of the pancreas, the mean coefficient of fat absorption was 80 per cent in the six patients who were thought to have had a 95 per cent pancreatic resection. The lipase concentration in the jejunum was 10 per cent of that in controls. One patient was estimated to have had a 75 per cent pancreatic resection, and fat absorption was normal.[97] Obstruction of the pancreatic ducts in rats resulted in absorption of 37 per cent of ^{14}C-labeled protein in a test meal. There was no detectable proteolytic activity in the lumen of the intestine. If the meal was introduced into a Thiry-Vella fistula of the small intestine, 30 per cent of the protein was absorbed in 4 hours. Predigesting the meal with acid-pepsin increased absorption to 50 per cent.[37] In dogs, ligation of either the pancreatic ducts or the common bile duct reduced fat absorption by 50 per cent, but ligation of both ducts did not reduce it further. In patients with pancreatic insufficiency there was no morphologic evidence of fat absorption, but 30 to 70 per cent of the fat was absorbed, as determined by balance studies.[171] Relief of surgical occlusion of pancreatic ducts in dogs 7 to 46 days later was followed initially by a period of reduced secretion of both bicarbonate and enzyme. A greater reduction in amylase secretion than in that of bicarbonate suggested either that the acinar cells are more sensitive to damage from obstruction or that the ductular cells have a greater regenerative capacity.[186]

A number of studies from Marseilles have suggested that the protein lactoferrin is present in increased amounts in the pancreatic juice and pancreatic tissue of patients with chronic pancreatitis, in proportion to the severity of the pancreatitis.[32, 58] While it does not appear to be the protein precipitated in the pancreatic ducts, it may serve as a marker to indicate that protein plugs are present.

There are other secretory abnormalities in the exocrine pancreas in chronic pancreatitis. Increased concentrations of calcium in the duodenal content are found after secretin stimulation. Calcium outputs may be unchanged by the decrease in volume.[201] The concentrations of serum immunoglobulins were also elevated in the 25 to 50 per cent of patients with chronic pancreatitis.[11] IgA was elevated in 50 per cent of 40 patients and IgA in 27.5 per cent. The IgA was not of the secretory type.[11] Basal outputs of bile acids in duodenal content were higher in patients with chronic pancreatitis. In response to alcohol administration by jejunal perfusion or intravenously, bile acid outputs decrease both in patients with pancreatitis and in normal controls

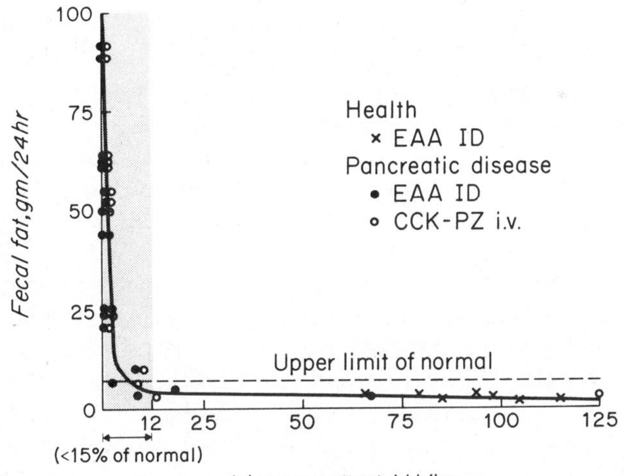

Figure 3–7. Relationship of pancreatic lipase outputs in duodenal content to 24-hour fecal fat excretion in healthy subjects and patients with chronic pancreatitis. Values above the horizontal dashed line equal steatorrhea (> 7 gm fat per 24 hours). The shaded area represents lipase outputs of less than 15 per cent of normal. EAA ID represents 78 mM essential amino acid mixture perfused into the duodenum at a rate of 10 ml per minute. CCK-PZ i.v. represents cholecystokinin-pancreozymin infused intravenously at a rate of 0.25 Crick-Harper-Raper unit per kilogram per minute while the duodenum is perfused with saline. (Reprinted, by permission, from DiMagno, E. P., Go, V. L. W., and Summerskill, W. H. J.: Relations between pancreatic enzyme outputs and malabsorption in severe pancreatic insufficiency. New Eng. J. Med. 288:814, 1973.)

when blood levels of alcohol reached 125 to 140 mg/100 ml.[117] The concentrations of ethanol were higher in bile than in plasma. Other investigators found normal outputs of bile acids after a meal but a lower than normal concentration and a smaller percentage in the micellar phase. Concentrations of bile lipids were also reduced and were related to the pH. These abnormalities could be corrected by a combination of cimetidine and viokase, suggesting that decreased secretion of pancreatic enzymes and bicarbonate was responsible.[147] The extent to which this phenomenon contributed to maldigestion of fat is not known.

The pathophysiology of the diabetic-type glucose intolerance in patients with chronic pancreatitis is not entirely clear. Overt diabetes is seen in about 70 per cent of patients with calcific pancreatitis and 30 per cent of those with noncalcific pancreatitis.[10] Plasma insulin levels rose from 25 to 155 μU 1 hour after glucose administration in two normal subjects but only from 9 to 64 μU in six patients with pancreatitis and diabetes. In four patients with pancreatitis without diabetes, the rise was normal. In eight patients with diabetes alone, the rise was from 40 to 321 μU/ml. Blood glucose rose similarly in the patients with pancreatitis and diabetes and in the patients with diabetes alone.[150] Plasma insulin rose from 30 to 310 μU/ml after administration of 100 gm of glucose in controls but only to 100 μU/ml in patients with chronic pancreatitis.[10] There is said to be less vascular disease in patients with chronic pancreatitis than in patients with diabetes mellitus.

Patients with juvenile-onset diabetes have decreased outputs of pancreatic enzymes and bicarbonate in response to administration of secretin-CCK.[45, 65] The decreases were unrelated to the duration of diabetes or the dose of insulin. There were no clinical signs of pancreatitis, and steatorrhea did not occur unless the patient had pancreatitis.

The malabsorption of chronic pancreatitis with steatorrhea is accompanied by increased urinary indican excretion. After a year of replacement therapy with pancreatic enzymes, the indican excretion returned to normal. It may be that partial digestion of protein is necessary if intestinal bacteria are to form indican.[122]

It has been noted that some patients with malabsorption associated with small bowel disease — e.g., celiac disease, Crohn's disease, blind loop syndromes, lymphoma, giardiasis, tuberculosis or folate deficiency — have decreased bicarbonate or amylase concentrations in duodenal content after secretin (Boots) stimulation. In one series of 50 patients with small bowel disease, 31 had values averaging 62 per cent of normal, but in only 6 patients was there moderate or severe pancreatic insufficiency.[133] A normal pancreas was verified by palpation at laparotomy in 32. The explanation for this is unknown. In preliminary studies with rather uncertain radioimmunoassays for

CCK, elevated values in chronic pancreatitis that might alter the response to exogenous hormone have been reported.[86a]

Clinically significant malabsorption of vitamin A with objective evidence of night blindness has been noted in patients with pancreatic insufficiency due to chronic pancreatitis.[189] The "brown bowel" syndrome, with pigment deposits in the wall of the intestine, is probably secondary to malabsorption of vitamin E. Osteolytic lesions of the long bones representing bone infarcts present dramatic roentgenologic changes but are usually asymptomatic. Diffuse osteomalacia and osteoporosis are uncommon. Hypoprothrombinemia with clinical evidence of bleeding is also unusual. These deficiencies of fat-soluble vitamins are presumably realted to steatorrhea and the malabsorption of fat, but zinc deficiency may contribute to night blindness.[189] Subclinical evidence of deficiency of fat-soluble vitamins is more common. On the basis of serum vitamin A levels, serum 25-hydroxy-vitamin D levels and a hemolysis test for vitamin E, deficiency of a single fat-soluble vitamin was found in 14 of 15 patients with pancreatic insufficiency, and 9 of 15 had deficiencies of two or more fat-soluble vitamins.[53]

About one third of patients with pancreatic insufficiency due to chronic pancreatitis have malabsorption of vitamin B_{12}, but pernicious anemia is rare.[190] The mechanism of malabsorption is still controversial. Both defective tryptic digestion and B_{12} binding factors have been implicated.[181, 191]

Reduced amounts of enterokinase, trypsin and disaccharidases were found in 14 infants with diarrhea and moderate degrees of intestinal mucosal injury, whereas in others with cystic fibrosis and the Shwachman-Diamond syndrome, enterokinase levels were normal or elevated.[105] Malabsorption of D-xylose, sodium and water but not glucose was demonstrated in patients with chronic pancreatitis only if steatorrhea was present.[89]

The levels of disaccharidases in the intestinal mucosa of patients with chronic pancreatitis have been reported to be elevated by some workers but not by others.[4, 114] Intestinal hormones may play a role in the pathophysiology of chronic pancreatitis: an increased level of immunoreactive (gastrointestinal inhibitory polypeptide) GIP after oral glucose was noted in patients with chronic pancreatitis and impaired glucose tolerance. The insulin release was below normal but levels of glucagon were elevated.[19] The increased GIP release may be secondary to low insulin levels. Glucagon levels were also higher than normal. The increase in pancreatic polypeptide in plasma after a meal was found to be decreased in patients with chronic pancreatitis but not in patients with recurrent pancreatitis.[195] Subsequently, impaired pancreatic polypeptide release was noted only in those patients with chronic pancreatitis and steatorrhea.[1] Recent studies found that an unknown factor present in crude CCK but not in the octapeptide markedly elevated serum pancreatic polypeptide levels in normal subjects.[144] Secretin administered intravenously increased pancreatic polypeptide release in normal subjects but not in patients with chronic pancreatitis and pancreatic insufficiency. Since pancreatic polypeptide is produced in the pancreas, this may merely reflect destruction of the cells that produce it.

No definite abnormalities in secretin release have been demonstrated in chronic pancreatitis, but one report of elevated fasting CCK levels has appeared that was based on an immunoassay that probably is not quantitatively precise.[86a]

Studies with homogenized fatty test meals indicated that patients with pancreatic insufficiency emptied the meal more rapidly from the stomach than did normal subjects and that this defect was corrected by adding pancreatic extracts to the meal.[111] More recently, using a gastroduodenal perfusion system, investigators found a decrease in gastric acid secretion during the first hour after the meal in patients with pancreatic insufficiency and a decrease in the amount of acid emptied. The total volume emptied was less than in normal subjects, but the fractional rate of emptying was the same. After 2 to 3 hours the pH of duodenal content was lower than normal. Fasting and postprandial serum gastrin levels were elevated.[146]

Since increased secretion of sodium and chloride in sweat is characteristic of cystic fibrosis, it has been of considerable interest to examine sweat electrolytes in chronic pancreatitis. By means of pilocarpine iontophoresis, 14 per cent of 84 patients with calcific pancreatitis and 6 per cent of 51 patients with noncalcific pancreatitis were found to have sweat chloride concentrations of greater than 120 mEq/L.[9] In one family with multiple members with chronic pancreatitis, 5 of 15 had chloride concentrations over 120 mEq/L. None of 37 adult controls had chloride concentrations over 120 mEq/L, and in only one did it reach 110 MEq/L. Another had a chloride concentration of 91 mEq/L. The significance of these observations is uncertain.

Our knowledge of the pathophysiology of chronic alcoholic pancreatitis in man is very scanty. The alcoholic intake of patients with chronic calcifying pancreatitis in Marseilles was 178 gm of pure ethanol per day, compared to 74 gm/day in controls matched for age, sex, race and profession.[156] In another series of 90 patients with chronic pancreatitis, alcohol intake was 129 gm/day. The diets of the patients were also richer in lipids and protein and higher in calories than those of normal controls.[156]

In 11 of 35 patients with pancreatitis, but in none of 25 controls, pancreatic juice obtained by direct cannulation of the duct by ERCP exhibited bacterial growth. The bile in four of six patients with pancreatitis also grew bacteria. The organisms were gram-negative and polymicrobial.[74]

ANIMAL MODELS OF CHRONIC PANCREATITIS

Two models of chronic alcoholic pancreatitis in animals have been developed in Sarles's laboratory. The daily administration to rats of 20 per cent ethanol for 20 to 30 months resulted in the development of lesions resembling those of human chronic pancreatitis in more than half the animals.[159] In experiments over 10 to 12 weeks of alcohol administration, the mitochondria of pancreatic acinar cells were found to become more easily disrupted[30] and the tryptic inhibitory activity of pancreatic juice was decreased.[94] After 8 months of alcohol administration, the concentration of protein in resting pancreatic juice was twice that in controls.[103] By 12 months it had returned to normal, but intragastric alcohol now increased protein output.[25, 103] Other investigators noted a decrease in output of total protein, while the output of active proteolytic enzymes increased.[91] The amount of trypsin inhibitors per milligram of protein in pancreatic juice decreased with stimulation by CCK and secretin. There was no change in the volume response to CCK.[93]

The effects of ethanol given to relatively small numbers of dogs over 21 to 34 months produced dilatation of the pancreatic ducts, protein plugs and periductal fibrosis.[163] A large number of publications from the same laboratory have explored various aspects of pancreatic exocrine secretion during chronic alcohol ingestion. The initial effect of alcohol was to decrease the volume of pancreatic juice secreted in response to secretin.[165] By 4 months this had reversed, and the volume increased above that in control dogs.[164] Earlier, at 6 weeks, the dogs had developed protein plugs and microstones in their ducts.[165] The protein response to CCK also increased at 4 months, as did that to a protein meal. At 8 months, the dogs showed a reduced volume and electrolyte response, but the protein concentration in pancreatic juice had increased 74 per cent and all three dogs secreted protein plugs.[188] The same investigators have reported decreased release of immunoreactive secretin in response to intraduodenal hydrochloric acid but higher gastrin levels in the blood after a meal in dogs given alcohol chronically.[22, 192] The fact that atropine inhibited the increased pancreatic secretory response in dogs on long-term alcohol intake but vagotomy did not suggested a role for cholinergic activity in the increased secretion during chronic alcohol ingestion.[187] Atropine also inhibited the increased secretory response to oleic acid in the duodenum.[197] There is histochemical evidence of increased numbers of cholinergic nerves in the same dogs. Therefore, abnormalities of both hormonal and nervous control systems of the pancreas occur with chronic alcohol administration in dogs, but their relationship to the histopathologic lesions in the pancreas remains unclear.

A decrease in bile flow in response to intravenous alcohol administration has been reported in chronic alcoholic dogs, while bile acid concentrations and outputs increased. In normal dogs, bile acid secretion decreased after alcohol administration.[55]

Dogs may develop pancreatic insufficiency spontaneously, and increased activities of selected brush border disaccharidases have been demonstrated in the jejunal mucosa, while the enterokinase and alkaline phosphatase levels remained normal.[13]

Recently a model of pancreatic insufficiency has been reported in the mouse. Mice of CBA/J strain were found to lack pancreatic acinar cells. Early in the course, the pancreatic tissue levels of trypsin and chymotrypsin were found to be increased. Subcellular fractions showed increased activity, and the trypsinogen of zymogen granules showed an enhanced susceptibility to autoactivation. The latter could be delayed by trypsin inhibitor. The genetic predisposition of CBA/J mice to the exocrine pancreatic insufficiency syndrome may be due to an enhanced susceptibility of trypsinogen to autoactivation. This in turn could be the result of inadequate levels of trypsin inhibitor or heparin sulfate in zymogen granules.[38]

Intestinal washings contained proteolytic activity less than one tenth that of controls, and no fecal tryptic activity could be detected.[101, 107] The disaccharidase activity of brush border intestinal preparations was increased in the proximal small intestine, but enterokinase levels were one tenth of normal.[101] Feeding pancreatic enzymes partially restored enzyme levels to normal.[101, 107]

In summary, it appears possible to simulate the chronic pancreatic insufficiency of man in animals, but no animal model is available that follows the course of chronic or chronic relapsing pancreatitis as seen in man.

ETIOLOGY OF CHRONIC PANCREATITIS

In the United States, it has been estimated that chronic alcoholism accounts for chronic relapsing pancreatitis in 90 per cent of the patients.[120] In the Cape Peninsula in South Africa, alcoholism accounts for 62 per cent of the cases of chronic pancreatitis.[118] In England, a retrospective study of 32 patients with chronic pancreatitis concluded that the cause was alcoholism in 17, biliary tract disease in 8, hyperlipidemia in 3, and hyperparathyroidism in 2.[143] A preliminary study of 90 unrelated patients with chronic alcoholic pancreatitis compared with 523 blood donors showed a significant increase in the HLA antigen BW-40 in the former. Both BW-40 and A-1 were more frequent in noncalcifying than in calcifying pancreatitis. There was no increase in the antigen in the patients with pancreatitis and diabetes.[70]

Other evidence for genetic factors in chronic pancreatitis comes from the study of patients with hereditary pancreatitis. In the United

States, this entity has been estimated to account for 1 per cent of the cases of chronic pancreatitis.[120] Examples have been followed through four generations.[76] The mode of inheritance has not been clear, but in a British family it was compatible with autosomal dominance with limited penetrance. None of those patients had aminoaciduria but half of another kindred had lysinuria and cystinuria. A defect in renal tubular reabsorption was demonstrated.[77] Glycinuria has also been found.[14] In a family studied recently with ERCP, demonstration of a markedly dilated duct with a "chain of lakes" appearance led the authors to raise the question of an inherited abnormality in the sphincter of Oddi.[116]

ERCP studies have suggested that a divided pancreas with a portion drained by the accessory duct of Santorini may be an important factor in pancreatitis of young persons who do not abuse alcohol.[34, 35]

Nutritional deficiency of the protein-calorie type can cause pancreatic insufficiency and atrophy. In Uganda it is a significant cause of pancreatic calcification. Among 36 patients, 17 had diabetes and 5 had a malabsorption syndrome. Abdominal pain was present in 18.[168] Kwashiorkor was associated with acinar cell atrophy and decrease in secretory granules determined by light microscopy in 14 children coming to autopsy.[16] Electron microscopy showed a diminished amount of rough endoplasmic reticulum, large mitochondria and an increase in the number of pores in the nuclear membrane. Patients on a low-food intake for 3 to 12 months have low volume and low bicarbonate and enzyme output in response to administration of CCK and secretin.[40] These return to normal with refeeding.

Schistosomiasis is a cause of pancreatitis in Brazil. It was found in the course of splenectomy and splenorenal shunts in 20 patients with portal hypertension and *Schistosoma mansoni* infestation. A lower than normal bicarbonate concentration in duodenal content after secretin stimulation was noted in 16 of the patients. The pancreatitis was localized to the tail of the pancreas histologically in 14 of the patients.[129]

Sjögren's syndrome has been reported in association with decreased pancreatic secretory function. Antibodies to pancreatic ductal cells were found in the serum of 4 of 12 patients, as well as in that of 8 of 31 patients with rheumatoid arthritis,[112] as demonstrated by cytoplasmic immunofluorescence.

SCREENING FOR CHRONIC PANCREATITIS

There is no satisfactory screening technique for chronic pancreatitis. When steatorrhea is present, a survey film of the abdomen is likely to show pancreatic calcification, but this is a late stage of the disease. Demonstration of a pseudocyst by ultrasonography may become a useful screening procedure in patients with pain suggestive of chronic pancreatic disease, but the value of ultrasonography and CAT scans in detecting abnormalities in the size of the pancreas remains to be seen.

PREVENTION OF CHRONIC PANCREATITIS

The obvious approach to the prevention of chronic pancreatitis is the prevention of chronic alcoholism, but this does not seem to be a likely route to success unless some means can be found to detect among chronic alcoholics a subset who are at particularly high risk. The detection and appropriate management of gallstone disease is perhaps more hopeful. It remains to be seen whether seat belts and the reduction of the speed limit will reduce the incidence of traumatic pancreatitis. Early detection and genetic counseling in hereditary pancreatitis may help.

REFERENCES

1. Adrian, T. E., Besterman, H. S., Mallinson, C. N., Geralotis, C., and Bloom, S. R.: Impaired pancreatic polypeptide release in chronic pancreatitis with steatorrhea. Gut 20:98–101, 1979
2. Ammann, R. W., Largiader, F., and Akovbiantz, A.: Pain relief by surgery in chronic pancreatitis. Scand. J. Gastroenterol. 14:209–215, 1979
3. Arvanitakis, C., and Cooke, A. R.: Diagnostic tests of exocrine pancreatic function and disease. Gastroenterology 74:932–948, 1978
4. Arvanitakis, C., and Olsen, W. A.: Intestinal mucosal disaccharidases in chronic pancreatitis. Am. J. Dig. Dis. 19:417–422, 1974
5. Ashton, M. G., Axon, A. T. R., and Lintott, D. J.: Lundh test and ERCP in pancreatic disease. Gut 19:910–915, 1978
6. Bachrach, W. H., Birsner, J. W., Izenstark, J. L., and Smith, V. L.: Pancreatic scanning: A review. Gastroenterology 63:890–910, 1972
7. Bank, S., Marks, I. N., and Kramer, I.: Isoenzymes of amylase in chronic pancreatitis. Gastroenterology 74:1005, 1978
8. Bank, S., Marks, I. N., Moshal, M. G., Efron, G., and Silber, R.: The pancreatic function test; method and normal values. S. Afr. Med. J. 37:1061–1066, 1963
9. Bank, S., Marks, I. N., and Novis, B.: Sweat electrolytes in chronic pancreatitis. Am. J. Dig. Dis. 23:178–181, 1978
10. Bank, S., Marks, I. N., and Vinik, A. I.: Clinical and hormonal aspects of pancreatic diabetes. Am. J. Gastroenterol. 64:13–22, 1975
11. Bank, S., Novis, B. H., Petersen, E., Dowdle, E., and Marks, I. N.: Serum immunoglobulins in calcific pancreatitis. Gut 14:723–725, 1973
12. Barnes, A. J., Bloom, S. R., George, K., Alberti, M. M., Smythe, P., Alford, F. P., and Chisholm, D. J.: Ketoacidosis in pancreatectomized man. New Eng. J. Med. 296:1250–1253, 1977
13. Batt, R. M., Nicholson, J. A., Bush, B. M., and Peters, T. J.: The effects of exocrine pancreatic insufficiency on the subcellular biochemistry of the jejunal mucosa — a naturally occurring model in the dog. Gastroenterology 76:1096, 1979
14. Bergstrom, K., Hellstrom, K., Kallner, M., and Lundh, G.: Familial pancreatitis associated with hyperglycinuria. Scand. J. Gastroenterol. 3:217–224, 1973

15. Berk, J. E., Ayulo, J. A., and Fridhandler, L.: Value of pancreatic-type isoamylase as an index of pancreatic insufficiency. Digest. Dis. Sci. 24:6–10, 1979

16. Blackburn, W. R., and Vinychaikul, K.: The pancreas in kwashiorkor. An electron microscopic study. Lab. Invest. 20:305–318, 1969

17. Bloom, S. R., Adrian, T. E., Besterman, H. S., Mallinson, C. N., and Geralotis, C.: Plasma trypsin in the diagnosis of steatorrhea due to chronic pancreatitis: RIA for plasma trypsin. Gastroenterology 74:1112, 1978

18. Bordalo, O., Noronha, M., Lamy, J., and Dreiling, D. A.: Standard and augmented secretin testing in chronic pancreatic alcoholic disease. Am. J. Gastroenterol. 64:25–132, 1975

19. Botha, J. L., Vinik, A. I., and Brown, J. C.: Gastric inhibitory polypeptide (GIP) in chronic pancreatitis. J. Clin. Endocrinol. Metab. 42:791–797, 1976

20. Braganza, J., Critchley, M., Howat H. T., Testa, H. J., and Torrance, H. B.: An evaluation of ^{75}Se selenomethionine scanning as a test of pancreatic function compared with the secretin-pancreozymin test. Gut 14:383–389, 1973

21. Braganza, J. M., Herman, K., Hine, P., Kay, G., and Sandle, G. I.: Pancreatic enzymes in human duodenal juice — a comparison of responses in secretin pancreozymin and Lundh-Borgstrom tests. Gut 19:358–366, 1978

22. Bretholz, A., Levesque, D., Viorol, M., Tiscornia, O. M., Bloom, S. R., and Sarles, H.: Impaired secretin release in chronic alcoholic dogs. Digestion 17:437–440, 1978

23. Buscharth, F., and Kam-Hansen, L.: Obstructive jaundice in pancreatitis investigated by percutaneous transhepatic cholangiography. Scand. J. Gastroenterol. 13:589–591, 1978

24. Cameron, J. L.: Chronic pancreatic ascites and pancreatic plural effusions. Gastroenterology 74:134–140, 1978

25. Carvarson, A., Teixeira, A., Sarles, H., and Tiscornia, O.: Action of intragastric ethanol on the pancreatic secretion of conscious rats. Digestion 13:145–152, 1975

26. Cavallini, G., Mirachian, R., Angelini, G., Vantini, I., Vaona, B., Bovo, P., Gelpi, F., Ederle, A., Dobrilla, G., and Scuro, L. A.: The role of the caerulein in tests of exocrine pancreatic function. Scand. J. Gastroenterol. 13:3–15, 1978

27. Cerda, J. J., and Brooks, F.P.: Relationships between steatorrhea and an insufficiency of pancreatic secretion in the duodenum in patients with chronic pancreatitis. Am. J. Med. Sci. 253:38–44, 1967

28. Christensen, B. C.: Studies on the secretin test. Acta Med. Scand. 173:315–327, 1963

29. Clain, J., Bank, S., Barbezat, G. O., Novis, B. H., and Marks, I. N.: A comparison between secretion alone and sequential and simultaneous secretin and cholecystokinin administration in the assessment of pancreatic function. Gut 15:885–888, 1974

30. Clemente, F., Durand, S.,, Laval, J., Thouvenot, J.-P., and Ribet, A.: Métabolisme de l'éthanol par le pancréas de rat. Gastroenterol. Clin. Biol. 1:39–48, 1977

31. Cohen, M. M., and Cooperberg, P. L.: Percutaneous fine needle pancreatography. Gastroenterology 76:1114, 1979

32. Colomb, E.,Pianetta, C., Estevenon, J. P., Guy, O., Figarella, C., and Sarles, H.: Lactoferrin in human pancreas. Immunohistological localization in normal and pathological pancreatic tissues. Digestion 14:242–249, 1976

33. Cotton, P. B.: Progress report. Cannulation of the papilla of Vater by endoscopy and retrograde cholangiopancreatography. Gut 13:1014–1025, 1972

34. Cotton, P. B.: Pancreas divisium — a new cause for pancreatic pain and recurrent pancreatitis. Gastroenterology 76:1116, 1979

35. Cotton, P. B., Denyer, M. E., Kreel, L., Husband, J., Meire, H. B., and Lees, W.: Comparative clinical impact of endoscopic pancreatography, grey-scale ultrasonography, and computed tomography (EMI scanning) in pancreatic disease: Preliminary report. Gut 19:679–684, 1978

36. Crozier, R. E.: The secretin test: Its shortcomings as a practical clinical diagnostic procedure. Lahey Clin. Found. Bull. 19:17–21, 1970

37. Curtis, K. L., Gaines, H. D., and Kim, Y. S.: Protein digestion and absorption in rats with pancreatic duct occlusion. Gastroenterology 74:1271–1276, 1978

38. Dempsey, E. C.: Premature intracellular activation of zymogens: A biochemical basis for the exocrine pancreatic insufficiency (EPI) syndrome in CBA/J mice. Gastroenterology 74:1172, 1978
39. Denyer, M. E., and Cotton, P. B.: Pure pancreatic juice studies in normal subjects and patients with chronic pancreatitits. Gut 20:89–97, 1979
40. Descos, L., Duclieu, J., and Minaire, Y.: Exocrine pancreatic insufficiency and primitive malnutrition. Digestion 15:90–95, 1977
41. DiMagno, E. P., and Go, V. L. W.: Exocrine pancreatic insufficiency: Current concepts of pathophysiology. Postgrad. Med. 52:135–144, 1972
42. DiMagno, E. P., Go, V. L. W., and Summerskill, W. H. J.: Relations between pancreatic enzyme outputs and malabsorption in severe pancreatic insufficiency. New Eng. J. Med. 288:813–815, 1973
43. DiMagno, E. P., Malagelada, J. R., Go, V. L. W., and Moertel, C. G.: Fate of orally ingested enzymes in pancreatic insufficiency. New Eng. J. Med. 296:1318–1322, 1977
44. Dixon, J. A., and Englert, E., Jr.: Growing role of early surgery in chronic pancreatitis: A practical clinical approach. Gastroenterology 61:375–381, 1971
45. Domschke, W., Tympner, F., Domschke, S., and Demling, L.: Exocrine pancreatic function in juvenile diabetics. Am.J. Dig. Dis. 20:309–312, 1975
46. Donowitz, M., Kerstein, M. D., and Spiro, H. M.: Pancreatic ascites. Medicine 53:183–195, 1974
47. Dreiling, D. A.: Pancreatic secretory testing in 1974. Gut 16:653–656, 1975
48. Dreiling, D. A., Greenstein, A. J., and Bordalo, O.: The hypersecretory states of the pancreas. Am. J. Gastroenterol. 59:505–511, 1973
49. Dreiling, D. A., and Soto, J. M.: The pancreatic involvement in disseminated "collagen" disorders. Am. J. Gastroenterol. 66:546–553, 1976
50. Drummey, G. D., Benson, J. A., and Jones, C. M.: Microscopical examination of the stool for steatorrhea. New Eng. J. Med. 264:85–88, 1961
51. Durr, H. K., Bindrich, D., and Bode, J. Ch.: The frequency of macroamylasemia and the diagnostic value of the amylase to creatinine ratio in patients with elevated serum amylase activity. Scand. J. Gastroenterol. 12:701–705, 1977
52. Durr, H. K., Otte, M., Forell, M. M., and Bodi, J. C.: Fecal chymotrypsin: A study of its diagnostic value by comparison with the secretin-cholecystokinin test. Digestion 17:404–409, 1978
53. Dutta, S. K., Costa, B. S., Russell, R. M., and Connor, T. B.: Fat-soluble vitamin deficiency in treated patients with pancreatic insufficiency. Gastroenterology 76:1126, 1979
54. Dutta, S, K., Mobrahan, S., and Iber, F. L.: Associated liver disease in alcoholic pancreatitis. Am. J. Dig. Dis. 23:618–622, 1978
55. Dzieniszewski, J., Tiscornia, O. M., Palasciano, G., Domingo, N., and Sarles, H.: The effects of acute and chronic ethanol administration on canine bile and exocrine pancreatic secretion., Am. J. Dig. Dis. 21:1037–1043, 1976
56. Eaton, S. B., Jr., and Ferrucci, J. T., Jr.: Radiology of the Pancreas and Duodenum. Philadelphia, W. B. Saunders Co., 1973, 399 pp.
57. Escourrow, J., Frexinos, J., and Ribet, A.: Biochemical studies of pancreatic juice collected by duodenal aspiration and endoscopic cannulation of the main pancreatic duct. Am. J. Dig. Dis. 23:173–177, 1978
58. Estevenon, J. P., Sarles, H., and Figarella, C.: Lactoferrin in the duodenal juice of patients with chronic calcifying pancreatitis. Scand. J. Gastroenterol. 10:327–330, 1975
59. Evans, W. B., and Wollaeger, E. E.: Incidence and severity of nutritional deficiency states in chronic exocrine pancreatic insufficiency: Comparison with nontropical sprue. Am. J. Dig. Dis. 11:594–606, 1966
60. Ferrucci, J. T.: Body ultrasonography. New Eng. J. Med. 300:538–542, 590–602, 1979
61. Ferrucci, J. T., Wittenberg, J., Black, E. B., Kirkpatrick R. H., and Hall, D. A.: Computed body tomography in chronic pancreatitis. Radiology 130:175–182, 1979
62. Figarella, C., DeCaro, A., Oi, I., and Sahel, J.: Lipase activity in blood following endoscopic pancreatography: Demonstration of its pancreatic origin and

existence of ductal or acino-venous pathways in man. Scand J. Gastroenterol. 13:393–399, 1978

63. Fontana, G., Bolondi, L., Conti, M., Plicchi, G., Gallo, L., Caletti, G. C., and Labo, G.: An evaluation of echography in the diagnosis of pancreatic disease. Gut 17:228–234, 1976

64. Freeman, H. J., Weinstein, W. M., Shnitka, T. K., Crockford, P. M., and Herbert, F. A.: Alpha-antitrypsin deficiency and pancreatic fibrosis. Ann. Intern. Med. 85:73–76, 1976

65. Frier, B. M., Saunders, J. H. B., Wormsley, K. G., and Bouchier, I. A. D.: Exocrine pancreatic function in juvenile-onset diabetes mellitus. Gut 17:685–691, 1976

66. Galmiche, J-P., Mallet, E., Colin, R., Reumont, G., and Geffroy, Y.: Résultats du dosage de la parathormone sérique immuno-réactive au cours des pancréatites de l'adult. Étude prospective de 40 malades. Gastroenterol. Clin. Biol. 1:653–660, 1977

67. Gaskin, K. J., Durie, P. R., Lee, L., and Forstner, G. C.: Co-lipase (CL) in pancreatic insufficiency (PI). Gastroenterology 76:1137, 1979

68. Goebell, H., Bode, Ch., Lepler, U., and Martini, G. A.: Funktionsuntersurchungen des exokrinen Pankreas bei leberzirrhosen verschiedener Atiologie, Hamochromatose und nach portokavalem Shunt. Acta Hepatosplenol. 18:437–452, 1971

69. Goldberg, G. M., Sale, J. K., Fawcett, N., and Wormsley, K. G.: Trypsin and chymotrypsin as aids in the diagnosis of pancreatic disease. Am. J. Dig. Dis. 17:780–792, 1972

70. Gosselin, M., Fauchet, R., Genetet, B., and Gastard, J.: Les antigènes HLA dans la pancréatite chronique alcoolique. Gastroenterol. Clin. Biol. 2:883–886, 1978

71. Grabner, W., Phillip, J., and Strigl, P.: The diagnostic value of oral glucose tolerance test and combined B-cell stimulation in chronic pancreatitis. Am. J. Dig. Dis. 18:1055–1060, 1973

72. Graham, D. Y.: Enzyme replacement therapy of exocrine pancreatic insufficiency in man. New Eng. J.Med. 296:1314–1317, 1977

73. Gregg, J. A., and Sharma, M. M.:Pancreatic hypersecretion in liver disease. Am. J. Dig. Dis. 23:9–11, 1978

74. Gregg, J. A.: Detection of bacterial infection of the pancreatic ducts in patients with pancreatitis and pancreatic cancer during endoscopic cannulation of the pancreatic duct. Gastroenterology 73:1005–1007, 1977

75. Gregg, J. A., and Sharma, M. M.: Endoscopic measurement of pancreatic juice secretory flow rates and pancreatic secretory pressures after secretin administration in human controls and in patients with acute relapsing pancreatitis, chronic pancreatitis and pancreatic cancer. Am. J. Surg. 136:569–574, 1978

76. Gross, J. B., Gambill, E. E., and Ulrich, J. A.: Hereditary pancreatitis. Description of a fifth kindred and summary of clinical features. Am. J. Med. 33:358–364, 1962

77. Gross, J. B., Ulrich, J. A., Jones, J. D., and Maher, F. T.: Endogenous renal clearances of 12 individual amino acids in 4 apparently healthy subjects and in 4 aminoaciduric persons of a kindred with hereditary pancreatitis. J. Lab. Clin. Med. 63:933–944, 1964

78. Guillemin, G., Cuilleret, J., Michel, A., Berard, P., and Feroldi, J.: Chronic relapsing pancreatitis: Surgical management including sixty-three cases of pancreaticoduodenectomy. Am. J. Surg. 122:802–807, 1971

79. Gullo, L., Costa, P. L., Fontana, G., and Labo, G.: Investigation of exocrine pancreatic function by continuous infusion of caerulein and secretin in normal subjects and in chronic pancreatitis. Digestion 14:97–107, 1976

80. Gutierrez, L. V., and Baron, J. H.: A comparison of Boots and GIH secretin as stimuli of pancreatic secretion in human subjects with or without chronic pancreatitis. Gut 13:721–725, 1972

81. Gyr, K., Agrawal, N. M., Felsenfeld, O., and Font, R. G.: Comparative study of secretin and Lundh meals. Am. J. Dig. Dis. 20:506–512, 1975

82. Haaga, J. R., Alfidi, R. J., Zelch, M. G., Meany, T. F., Boller, M., Gonzalez, G., and Jelden, G. L.: Computed tomography of the pancreas. Radiology, 120:589–595, 1976

83. Hadorn, B.: The exocrine pancreas. *In* Paediatric Gastroenterology, edited by C. M. Anderson and V. Burke, Oxford, Blackwell Scientific Publications, 1975, pp. 289–327

84. Hansky, J.: Pancreatic function tests: Comparison of standard and augmented secretin. Aust. N. Z. J. Med. 1:109–113, 1971

85. Hanssen, L. E., Osnes, M., and Myren, J.: Pancreatic secretion obtained by endoscopic cannulation of the main pancreatic duct and secretin release after duodenal acidification in man. Scand. J. Gastroenterol. 13:325–330, 1978

86. Hartley, R. C., Gambill, E E., Engstrom, G. W., and Summerskill, W. H. J.: Pancreatic exocrine function. Comparison of responses to augmented secretin stimulus, augmented pancreozymin stimulus, and test meal in health and disease. Am. J. Dig. Dis. 11:27–39, 1966

86a. Harvey, R. F., Rey, J. F., Howard, J. M., Read, A. E., Groarke, J. F., Fitzgerald, O., Ederle, A. and Vantini, I.: Serum cholecystokinin in pancreatic disase. Gut 17:827, 1976

87. Hegarty, J. E., O'Donnell, M. D., McGeeney, K. F., and Fitzgerald, O.: Pancreatic and salivary amylase/creatinine clearance ratios in normal subjects and in patients with chronic pancreatitis. Gut 19:350–354, 1978

88. Heizer, W. D., Cleaveland, C. R., and Iber, F. L.: Gastric inactivation of pancreatic supplements. Bull. Johns Hopkins Hosp. 116:261–270, 1965

89. Helman, C. A., Barbezat, G. O., and Bank, S.: Jejunal monosaccharide water and electrolyte transport in patients with chronic pancreatitis. Gut 19:46–49, 1978

90. Howard, J. M., and Nedwich, A.: Correlation of the histologic observations and operative findings in patients with chronic pancreatitis. Surg. Gynecol. Obstet. 132:387–395, 1971

91. Huttunen, R., Huttunen, P., and Jalovaara, P.: The effect of chronic intragastric alcohol ingestion on the pancreatic secretion of the rat. Scand. J. Gastroenterol. 11:103–106, 1976

92. Ihse, I., Arnesjo, B., Kugelberg, C., and Lilja, P.: Intestinal activities of trypsin, lipase and phospholipase after a test meal. An evaluation of 474 examinations. Scand. J. Gastroenterol. 12:663–668, 1977

93. Jalovaara, P.: Pancreatic exocrine secretion in the rat after chronic alcohol ingestion: Nonparallel secretion of proteins and pancreatic secretory trypsin inhibitor. Scand. J. Gastroenterol. 14:57–63, 1979

94. Jalovaara, P., and Huttunen, R.: The effect of chronic ethanol ingestion on the pancreatic proteolytic enzymes and their inhibitors in the rat. Scand. J. Gastroenterol. 12:785–792, 1977

95. Jimenez, H., and Aldrete, J. S.: Analysis of 101 cases of chronic pancreatitis with emphasis on the indications and results of its operative treatment. Gastroenterology 76:1161, 1979

96. Johnson, S. G., and Levitt, M. D.: Relation between serum pancreatic isoamylase concentration and pancreatic exocrine function. Am. J. Dig. Dis. 23:914–918, 1978

97. Kalser, M. H., Leite, C. A., and Warren, W. D.: Fat assimilation after massive distal pancreatectomy. New Eng. J. Med. 279:570–576, 1968

98. Kotler, D. P., and Levine, G. M.: Reversible gastric and pancreatic hyposecretion after long term total parenteral nutrition. New Eng. J. Med. 300:241–242, 1979

99. Kruse, A., Thommesen, P., and Frederiksen, P.: Endoscopic retrograde cholangiopancreatography in pancreatic cancer and chronic pancreatitis — differences in morphologic changes in the pancreatic duct and the bile duct. Scand. J. Gastroenterol. 13:513–518, 1978

100. Kugelberg, C. H., Wehlin, L., Arnesjo, B., and Tylen, U.: Endoscopic pancreatography in evaluating results of pancreatico-jejunostomy. Gut 17:267–272, 1976

101. Kwong, W. K. L., Seetharam, B., and Alpers, D. H.: Effect of exocrine pancreatic insufficiency on small intestine in the mouse. Gastroenterology 74:1277–1282, 1978

102. Lagerlof, H. D.: Pancreatic secretion: Pathophysiology. *In* Handbook of Physiology, Section 6, Alimentary Canal, Vol. II, Secretion, edited by C. F. Code. Washington, American Physiological Society, 1967, pp. 1027–1042

103. Langier, R., and Sarles, H.: Effets de la consommation chronique d'alcool sur la sécretion pancrêatique exocrine du rat. Variations en function de la duré de consommation. Gastroenterol. Clin. Biol. 1:767–774, 1977

104. Lawson, T. L.: Sensitivity of pancreatic ultrasonography in the detection of pancreatic disease. Radiology 128:733–736, 1978

105. Lebenthal, E., Antonowicz, I., and Shwachman, H.: Enterokinase and trypsin activities in pancreatic insufficiency and diseases of the small intestine. Gastroenterology 70:508–512, 1976

106. Leger, L., Lenriot, J. P., and Lemaigre, G.: Five to 20-year follow-up after surgery for chronic pancreatitis in 148 patients. Ann. Surg. 180:185–191, 1974

107. Leiter, E. H., and Cunliffe-Beamer, T.: Exocrine pancreatic insufficiency syndrome in CBA/J mice. III. Pathological and genetic analysis. Gastroenterology 73:260–266, 1977

108. Levrat, M., Descos, L., Moulinier, B., and Pasquier, J.: Évolution au long cours des pancréatites chroniques. I. Étude de l'évolution spontanée. Arch. Fr. Mal. App. Dig. 59:5–18, 1970

109. Levarat, M., Descos, L., Moulinier, B., and Pasquier, J.: Évolution au long cours des pancréatites chroniques. II. Étude de l'évolution de la pancréatite chronique chez les malades operés. Arch. Fr. App. Dig. 59:305–314, 1970

110. Linde, J. H., Nilsson, H. S., and Barany, F. R.: Diabetes and hypoglycemia in chronic pancreatitis. Scand. J. Gastroenterol. 12:369–373, 1977

111. Long, W. B., and Weiss, J. B.: Rapid gastric emptying of fatty meals in pancreatic insufficiency. Gastroenterology 67:920–925, 1974

112. Ludwig, H., Schernthaner, G., Scherak, O., and Kolarz, G.: Antibodies to pancreatic duct cells in Sjogren's syndrome and rheumatoid arthritis. Gut 18:311–315, 1977

113. Lurie, B., Brom, B., Bank, S., Novis, B., and Marks, I. N.: Comparative response of exocrine pancreatic secretion following a test meal and secretin-pancreozymin stimulation. Scand. J. Gastroenterol. 8:27–32, 1973

114. Machado, W. M., Bettarello, A., Mott, C. B., and Fibo, J. M.: Presented at the 26th Brazilian Congress of Gastroenterology, Curitiba, Brazil, April 30–May 4, 1979

115. Magdid, E., Hersing, M., and Rune, S. J.: On the quantitation of isoamylases in serum and the diagnostic value of serum pancreatic-type amylase in chronic pancreatitis. Scand. J. Gastroenterol. 12:621–628, 1977

116. Malik, S. A., VanKley, H., and Knight, W. A.: Inherited defect in hereditary pancreatitis. Am. J. Dig. Dis. 22:999–1004, 1977

117. Marin, G. A., Ward, N. L., and Fischer, R.: Effect of ethanol on pancreatic and biliary secretions in humans. Am. J. Dig. Dis 18:825–833, 1973

118. Marks, I. N., Bank, S., and Louw, J. H.: Some current views of pancreatitis. S. Afr. Med. J. 45:1138–1140, 1971

119. McElroy, R., and Christiansen, P. A.: Hereditary pancreatitis in a kinship associated with portal vein thrombosis. Am. J. Med. 52:228–241, 1972

120. Mendeloff, A. I., and Dunn, J. P.: Digestive Diseases. Cambridge, Harvard University Press, 1971, pp. 105–113

121. Mezey, E., Jaw, E., Slavin, R. E., and Tobon, F.: Pancreatic function and intestinal absorption in chronic alcoholism. Gastroenterology 59:657–664, 1970.

122. Miloszewski, K., Kelleher, J., Walker, B. E., Davies, T., Smith, C. L., and Losowsky, M. S.: Increase in urinary indican excretion in pancreatic steatorrhea following replacement therapy. Scand. J. Gastroenterol. 10:481–486, 1975

123. Minaire, Y., and Descos, L.: Comparison of caerulein and cholecystokinin effects upon enzyme concentrations in duodenal aspirates. Digestion 15:86–89, 1977

124. Minaire, Y., Descos, L., Daly, J. P., Bererd, M. B., and Lambert, R.: The interrelationships of pancreatic enzymes in health and disease under cholecystokinin stimulation. Digestion 9:8–20, 1973

125. Moeller, D. D., Dunn, G. D., and Klotz, A. P.: Comparison of the pancreozymin secretin test and the Lundh test meal. Am. J. Dig. Dis. 17:799–805, 1972

126. Moeller, D. D., Dunn, G. D., and Klotz, A. P.: Diagnosis of pancreatic exocrine insufficiency by fecal chymotrypsin activity. Am. J. Dig. Dis. 18:792–796, 1973

127. Moore, J. G., Englert, E., Jr., Bigler, A. H., and Clark, R. W.: Simple fecal tests of absorption: A prospective study and technique. Am. J. Dig. Dis. 16:97–106, 1971

128. Moss, A. A., and Kressel, H. Y.: Computed tomography of the pancreas. Am. J. Dig. Dis. 22:1018–1027, 1977

129. Mott, C. B., Neves, D. P., Okumura, M., DeBrito, T., and Bettarello, A.: Histologic and functional alternations of human exocrine pancreas in Manson's schistosomiasis. Am. J. Dig. Dis. 17:583–590, 1972

130. Mottaleb, A., Kapp, F., Noguera, E. C. A., Kellock, T. D., Wiggins, H. S., and Waller, S. L.: The Lundh test in the diagnosis of pancreatic disease: A review of five years experience. Gut 14:835–841, 1973

131. Nakajima, S., Nakano, S., Horiguchi, Y., and Suzuki, T.: Relation of exocrine pancreatic function to the diameter of the pancreatic and common bile ducts. Am. J. Gastroenterol. 65:142–147, 1976

132. Nakamura, K., Sarles, H., and Payan, H.: Three-dimensional reconstruction of the pancreatic duct in chronic pancreatitis. Gastroenterology 62:942–949, 1972

133. Novis, B. H., Bank, S., and Marks, I. N.: Exocrine pancreatic function in intestinal malabsorption and small bowel disease. Am. J. Dig. Dis. 17:489–494, 1972

134. Osnes, M.,Petersen, H., and Schrumpf, E.: Comparison of juice obtained during duodenal aspiration and cannulation of the main pancreatic duct after stimulation with exogenous secretin in man. Scand. J. Gastroenterol. 13:453–458, 1978

135. O'Sullivan, J. N., Nobrega, F. T., Morlock, C. G., Brown, A. L., Jr., and Bartholomew, L. G.: Acute and chronic pancreatitis in Rochester, Minn., 1940–1969. Gastroenterology 62:373–379, 1972

136. Owyang, C., Miller, L. J., DiMagno, E. P., Mitchell, J. C., and Go, V. L. W.: Pancreatic exocrine function in human chronic renal failure. Gastroenterology 76:1213, 1979

137. Perman, G., and Bonera, E.: The secretin test in patients with hemochromatosis. Acta Med. Scand. 175:787–790, 1964

138. Petersen, H.: The duodenal aspirate following secretin stimulation — a variance study in man. Scand. J. Gastroenterol. 4:407–412, 1969

139. Petersen, H.: Bicarbonate and acid secretion in the diagnosis of pancreatic disease. Scand. J. Gastroenterol. 5:555–559, 1970

140. Petersen, H., and Berstad, A.: Comparison of response to intravenous injection of secretin in man. Scand. J. Gastroenterol. 7:463–469, 1972

141. Plessier, J., Lemonnier, F., Rubman, A., Troupel, S., Duhamel, F., Plessier, B., and Legousse, S.: Interêt de la double épreuve sécretine pancréozymine dans l'exploration functionelle du pancréas. Rev. Int. Hepatol. 13:491–510, 1963

142. Raffensperger, E. C., D'Agostino, F., Manfredo, H., Ramirez, M., Brooks, F. P., and O'Neill, F.: Fecal fat excretion. Arch. Intern. Med 119:573–576, 1967

143. Read, G., Braganza, J. M., and Howat, H. T.: Pancreatitis — a retrospective study. Gut 17:945–952, 1976

144. Regan, P. T., Go, V. L. W., and DiMagno, E. P.: Exocrine and endocrine pancreatic function in man in response to cholecystokinin (CCK) and octopeptide of CCK (CCK-OP). Gastroenterology 76:1224, 1979

145. Regan, P. T., Malagelada, J. R., DiMagno, E. P., Glanzman, S. L., and Go, V. L. W.: Comparative effects of antacids, cimetidine and enteric coating on the therapeutic response to oral enzymes in severe pancreatic insufficiency. New Engl. J. Med. 297:854–858, 1977

146. Regan, P. T., Malagelada, J. R., DiMagno, E. P., and Go, V. L. W.: Postprandial gastric function in pancreatic insufficiency. Gut 20:249–254, 1979

147. Regan, P. T., Malagelada, J. R., Go, V. L. W., and DiMagno, E. P.: The effect of treatment on abnormalities of intraluminal bile acid (BA) metabolism in pancreatic insufficiency (PI). Gastroenterology 74:1084, 1978

148. Renner, I. G., Rinderknecht, H., Valenzuela, J. E., and Douglas, A. P.: Abnormalities in pure pancreatic juice (PPJ) from human chronic alcoholics. Clin. Res. 26:112A, 1978

149. Ribet, A., Tournut, R., Duffaut, M., and Vaysse, N.: Use of caerulein with submaximal doses of secretin as a test of pancreatic function in man. Gut 17:431–434, 1976

150. Rogers, J. B., Howard, J. M., and Pairent, F. W.: Serum insulin levels in patients with chronic pancreatitis. Am. J. Surg. 119:171–176, 1970
151. Rolny, P., and Jagenburg, R.: The secretin-CCK test and a modified Lundh test. Scand. J. Gastroenterol. 13:927–931, 1978
152. Rolny, P., Lukes, P. J., Gamklou, R., Jagenburg, R., and Nilson, A.: A comparative evaluation of endoscopic retrograde pancreatography and secretin-CCK test in the diagnosis of pancreatic disease. Scand. J. Gastroenterol. 13:777–782, 1978
153. Rosch, J., and Bret, J.: Arteriography of the pancreas. Am. J. Roentgenol. 94:182–193, 1965
154. Russell, J. G. B., Vallan, A. G., Braganza, J. M., and Howat, H. T.: Ultrasonic scanning in pancreatic disease. Gut 19:1027–1033, 1978
155. Sahel, J., and Sarles, H.: Modification of pure human pancreatic juice induced by chronic alcohol consumption. Gastroenterology 76:1233, 1979
156. Sarles, H.: Alcoholism and pancreatitis. Scand. J. Gastroenterol. 6:193–198, 1971
157. Sarles, H.: Chronic calcifying pancreatitis — chronic alcoholic pancreatitis. Gastroenterology 66:604–616, 1974
158. Sarles, H., and Crousillat, B.: Fréquence des arteriopathies dans les pancréatites chroniques. Gastroenterol. Clin. Biol. 2:791–796, 1978
159. Sarles, H., Lebreuil, G., Tasso, F., Figarella, C., Clemente, F., Devaux, M. A., Fagonde, B., and Payan, H.: A comparison of alcoholic pancreatitis in rat and man. Gut 12:377–388, 1971
160. Sarles, H., Pastor, J., Pauli, A. M., and Barthelmy, M.: Determination of pancreatic function. Gastroenterologia 99:279–300, 1963
161. Sarles, H., and Sahel, J.: Pathology of chronic calcifying pancreatitis. Am. J. Gastroenterol. 66:117–139, 1976
162. Sarles, H., and Sahel, J.: Cholestasis and lesions of the biliary tract in chronic pancreatitis. Gut 19:851–857, 1978
163. Sarles, H., Sahel, J., Lebreuil, G., and Tiscornia, O. M.: Alcoholic experimental pancreatitis in dog. Pathological study. Biol. Gastroenterol. (Paris) 8:363, 1975
164. Sarles H., Tiscornia, O., and Palasciano, G.: Chronic alcoholism and canine exocrine pancreas secretion. Gastroenterology 72:238–243, 1977
165. Sarles, H., Tiscornia, O. M., Palasciano, G., Brosen, A. Hage, G., Devaux, M. A., and Gullo, L.: Effects of chronic intragastric ethanol administration on canine exocrine pancreatic secretion. Scand. J. Gastroenterol. 8:85–96, 1973
166. Saunders, J. H. B., and Wormsley, K. G.: Pancreatic extracts in the treatment of pancreatic exocrine insufficiency. Gut 16:157–162, 1975
167. Scott, J., Summerfield, A., Elias, E., Dick, R., and Sherlock, S.: Chronic pancreatitis: A cause of cholestasis. Gut 18:196–201, 1977
168. Shaper, A. G.: Aetiology of chronic pancreatic fibrosis with calcification seen in Uganda. Br. Med. J. 1:1607, 1964
169. Sheldon, W.: Congenital pancreatic lipase deficiency. Arch. Dis. Child. 39:268–271, 1964
170. Shichiri, M., Etani, N., Yoshida, M., Harano, U., Moshi, M., Shigeta, Y., and Abe, H.: Radio-selenium pancreozymin-secretin test as a clinical test for pancreatic exocrine function. Am. J. Dig. Dis. 20:460–468, 1975
171. Shimoda, S. S., Saunders, D. R., Schuffler, M. D., and Leinbach, G. L.: Electron microscopy of the small intestinal mucosa in pancreatic insufficiency. Gastroenterology 67:19–27, 1974
172. Sibert, J. R.: A British family with hereditary pancreatitis. Gut 16:81–88, 1975
173. Sileo, A. V., Chawla, S. K., and LoPresti, P. A.: Pancreatic ascites: Diagnostic importance of ascitic lipase. Am. J. Dig. Dis. 20:1110–1115, 1975
174. Simon, M., Gosselin, M., Kerbaol, M., Delanoe, G., Trebaul, L., and Bourel, M.: Functional study of exocrine pancreas in idiopathic hemochromatosis, untreated and treated by venesections. Digestion 8:485–496, 1973
175. Skude, G., and Eriksson, S.: Serum isoamylases in chronic pancreatitis. Scand. J. Gastroenterol. 11:525–528, 1976
176. Skude, G., and Ihse, I.: Salivary amylase in duodenal aspirates. Scand. J. Gastroenterol. 11:17–20, 1976

177. Skude, G., Wehlin, L., and Ohashi, K.: Serum isoamylase pattern in obstructive pancreatic disease. Scand. J. Gastroenterol. 12:673–676, 1977
178. Smith, F. R., Barkin, J. S., Perereas, R., Livingstone, A., and Rogers, A. I.: Therapeutic percutaneous aspiration of pancreatic pseudocysts. Gastroenterology 76:1250, 1979
179. Snape, W. J., Jr., Long, W. B., Trotman, B. W., Marin, G. A., and Czaja, A. J.: Marked alkaline phosphatase elevation with partial common bile duct obstruction due to calcific pancreatitis. Gastroenterology 70:70–73, 1976
180. Sottomayer, M., Chong, R. N., and Dawson, M.: Use of ERCP in the diagnosis of internal pancreatic fistula. Gut 19:244–246, 1978
181. Steinberg, W. M., Carrington, C. W., and Toskes, P. P.: Evidence that failure to degrade R-binder is unimportant in the pathogenesis of cobalamine malabsorption in patients with chronic pancreatitis. Gastroenterology 76:1255, 1979
182. Stone, L. B., Eaton, S. B., Jr., and Ferrucci, J. T., Jr.: Inflammatory disease of the pancreas. Curr. Probl. Radiol. 5:1–43, 1975
183. Strum, W. B., and Spiro, H. M.: Chronic pancreatitis. Ann. Intern. Med. 74:264–277, 1971
184. Tandon, B. N., George, P. K., Sama, S. K., Ramachandran, K., and Gandhi, P. C.: Exocrine pancreatic function in protein-calorie malnutrition disease of adults. Am. J. Clin. Nutr. 22:1476–1482, 1969
185. Thomas, E., Harkett, E. O., Halloran, M. W., Hislop, I. G., and Grant, A. K.: An evaluation of the secretin test in chronic pancreatic disease. Med. J. Aust. 11:860–863, 1972
186. Tiscornia, O. M., and Dreiling, D. A.: Recovery of pancreatic exocrine secretory capacity following prolonged ductal obstruction. Ann. Surg. 164:267–270, 1966
187. Tiscornia, O. M., Palasciano, G., and Sarles, H.: Atropine and exocrine pancreatic secretion in alcohol-fed dogs. Am. J. Gastroenterol. 63:33–36, 1975
188. Tiscornia, O. M., Singer, M., Mendes de Olivara, J. P., Demol, P., and Sarles, H.: Exocrine pancreas response to a test meal in the dog: Changes induced by 3 months' ethanol feeding. Am. J. Dig. Dis. 22:769–774, 1977
189. Toskes, P. P., Dawson, W., Carrington, C., Levy, N. S., and Fitzgerald, C.: Non-diabetic retinal abnormalities in chronic pancreatitis. New Eng. J. Med. 300:942–946, 1979
190. Toskes, P. P., Hansell, J., Cerda, J. J., and Deren, J. J.: Vitamin B_{12} malabsorption in chronic pancreatic insufficiency. New Eng. J. Med. 284:627–632, 1971
191. Toskes, P. P., Smith, G. W., Francis, G. M., and Sander, E. G.: Evidence that pancreatic proteases enhance vitamin B_{12} absorption by acting on crude preparation of hog intrinsic factor and human gastric juice. Gastroenterology 72:31–36, 1977
192. Treffot, M. J., Tiscornia, O. M., Palasciano, G., Hage, G., and Sarles, H.: Chronic alcoholism and endogenous gastrin. Am. J. Gastroenterol. 63:29–36, 1975
193. Tympner, F., and Rosch, W.: Pancreatic function test in patients with Billroth II resection with the aid of an endoscope. Endoscopy 6:245–247, 1974
194. Vagne, M., and Descos, L.: Pancreatic secretion of bicarbonate in patients with chronic pancreatitis. Digestion 3:350–356, 1970
195. Valenzuela, J. E., Taylor, I. L., and Walsh, J. H.: Pancreatic polypeptide (PP). Responses to a meal in pancreatitis. Gastroenterology 74:1149, 1978
196. Van der Hoeden, R., Wettendorff, P., and Delcourt, A.: Limits of the evocative pancreatic function test in the diagnosis of low-grade pancreatitis. Gut 14:763–766, 1973
197. Voirol, M., Bretholz, A., Levesque, R., Laugier, R., Tiscornia, O., and Sarles, H.: Atropine-induced inhibition of the enhanced CCK release observed in alcoholic dogs. Digestion 14:174–178, 1976
198. Warren, K. W., and Mountain, J. C.: Comprehensive management of chronic relapsing pancreatitis. Surg. Clin. North Am. 51:693–710, 1971
199. Warshaw, A. L., and Lee, K. H.: Aging changes of pancreatic isoamylases and the appearance of "old amylase" in the serum of patients with pancreatic pseudocysts. Gastroenterology 76:1266, 1979
200. Warshaw, A. L., Schapiro, R. H., Ferrucci, J. T., Jr., and Galdabini, J. J. Persistent obstructive jaundice, cholangitis, and biliary cirrhosis due to common bile duct stenosis in chronic pancreatitis. Gastroenterology, 70:562–567, 1976

201. Warwick, R. R. G., Tothill, P., Percy-Robb, I. W., and Shearman, D. J. C.: The calcium concentration in pancreatic secretion in chronic pancreatitis and carcinoma of the pancreas. Scand. J. Gastroenterol. 8:301–306, 1973
202. Way, L. W., Gadacz, T., and Goldman, L.: Surgical treatment of chronic pancreatitis. Am. J. Surg. 127:202–209, 1974
203. Waye, J. D., Adler, M., and Dreiling, D. A.: The pancreas: A correlation of function and structure. Am. J. Gastroenterol. 69:176–181, 1978
204. White, T. T., Elmslie, R. G., and Magee, D. F.: The disappearing enzymes. Am. J. Surg. 106:307–316, 1963
205. Wormsley, K. G.: A comparison of the response to secretin, pancreozymin and a combination of these hormones in man. Scand. J. Gastroenterol. 4:413–417, 1970
206. Wormsley, K. G.: Tests of pancreatic secretion. Clin. Gastroenterol. 7:529–544, 1978
207. Youngs, G. R., Agnew, J. E., Levin, G. E., and Bouchier, I. A. D.: A comparative study of 4 tests of pancreatic function in the diagnosis of pancreatic disease. Quart. J. Med. 42:597–618, 1973
208. Zeitlin, J. J., and Sircus, W.: Factors influencing duodenal trypsin levels following a standard test meal as a test of pancreatic function. Gut 15:173–179, 1974
209. Zieve, L., Silvis, S. E., Mulford, B., and Blackwood, W. D.: Secretion of pancreatic enzymes in response to secretin and pancreozymin. Am. J. Dig. Dis. 11:671–684, 1966

CHAPTER 4

CARCINOMA OF THE PANCREAS AND OTHER TUMORS OF THE EXOCRINE PANCREAS

Carcinoma is the most common tumor of the pancreas. In the last few years a variety of new diagnostic techniques have been introduced that are now undergoing evaluation. In addition, surgical techniques for radical removal are once again under consideration. Risk factors in pancreatic carcinoma and animal models are other areas of interest that are under active investigation. A National Pancreatic Cancer Study Group has been formed and has stimulated research in pancreatic cancer.

Another group of pancreatic exocrine neoplasms are the cystadenomas and cystadenocarcinomas. They are noteworthy because of their characteristic diagnostic features and because survival rates of patients with these tumors are better than those of patients with adenocarcinoma of the pancreas.

HOW THE PATIENT WITH PANCREATIC CARCINOMA PRESENTS

The clinical presentation of patients with carcinoma of the pancreas can be considered from four points of view: (1) analysis of all patients as seen originally for diagnosis; (2) analysis of patients with biopsy diagnoses or autopsy diagnoses; (3) analysis of symptoms in relation to the site of the tumor — e.g., head, body and tail; and (4) analysis according to a grouping of symptoms as clinical syndromes.

The most common presenting complaint of patients with carcinoma of the pancreas is pain (Table 4–1). In a large series of 239 patients from the Mayo Clinic, 64 per cent reported that pain was their first symptom of the disease.[34] In 56 per cent of patients, the pain was abdominal; in 31 per cent, it was in the back as a first symptom. Particularly late in the disease, the pain was usually constant rather than intermittent, often interfered with sleep and usually required salicylates or opiates rather than antacids for relief.[61] It is important to note that 20 per cent of patients complained of epigastric bloating rather than pain as the first symptom of pancreatic cancer. Most patients lost weight but it was not documented reliably as a first symptom. Anorexia or nausea was also the first symptom in 31 per cent of patients. Jaundice was a first symptom in only 10 per cent, dark urine in 6 per cent and pruritus in 5 per cent. Weakness or fatigue presented first in 17 per cent of patients.

Symptoms related to maldigestion and malabsorption were less frequent: diarrhea was a first symptom in 6 per cent, steatorrhea in only 2 per cent and constipation in 3 per cent of patients. Diabetes was the first complaint in 3 per cent. Systemic complaints such as fever were initial complaints in 3 per cent; chills were the first

*TABLE 4–1. FREQUENCY OF SYMPTOMS AND OCCURRENCE AS INITIAL SYMPTOMS IN CARCINOMA OF THE PANCREAS**

	SYMPTOM		INITIAL SYMPTOM	
	No.	%	No.	%
Pain	213	89	152	64
Abdominal	190	80	134	56
Back	139	58	74	31
Weight loss	161	67		
Anorexia and/or nausea	147	62	74	31
Jaundice	101	42	23	10
Subjective epigastric bloating	82	34	48	20
Weakness and/or fatigue	75	31	40	17
Diarrhea	60	25	22	9
Dark urine	60	25	15	6
Vomiting	54	23	15	6
Pruritus	42	18	12	5
Constipation	27	11	8	3
Steatorrhea	25	11	4	2
Fever	23	10	7	3
Diabetes	21	9	7	3
Upper GI bleed	18	8	6	3
Chills	14	6	4	2
Thrombophlebitis	8	3	0	
Depression	5	2	4	2
Dysphagia	3	1	0	
Coma	1			

*From Gambill, E. E.: Pancreatic and ampullary carcinoma: Diagnosis and prognosis in relationship to symptoms, physical findings, and elapse of time as observed in 255 patients. South. Med. J. 63:1120, 1970. Reprinted by permission from The Southern Medical Journal.

*TABLE 4-2.   PANCREATIC ADENOCARCINOMA (239 PATIENTS):
FREQUENCY AND ORDER OF APPEARANCE OF
ABDOMINAL PAIN**

			PATIENTS WITH PAIN AT SITE			
			Order of Appearance of Pain			
SITE OF PAIN	No.	*% of* 239	*1*	*2*	*3*	*4*
			Patients			
Midepigastrium	110	46	76 (32)†	23	9	2
Upper abdomen	55	23	31 (13)	18	6	0
Lower abdomen	47	20	27 (11)	16	3	1
Right upper quadrant	44	18	24 (10)	13	7	0
Left upper quadrant	30	13	16 (7)	9	4	1

*From Gambill, E. E.: Pancreatic and ampullary carcinoma: Diagnosis and prognosis in relationship to symptoms, physical findings and elapse of time as observed in 255 patients. South. Med. J. 63:1120, 1970. Reprinted by permission from The Southern Medical Journal.

†Number in parentheses is percent of 239 patients.

complaint in 2 per cent. In 3 per cent of patients, the first complaint was upper gastrointestinal hemorrhage. A summary of the incidence of various symptoms occurring at any time up to admission is also shown in Table 4–1.

The pain was initially localized to the midepigastrium in 32 per cent, to the upper abdomen in 13 per cent and to the lower abdomen in 11 per cent. In 10 per cent it was located in the right upper quadrant and in 7 per cent in the left upper quadrant (Table 4–2). In the case of back pain as the initial symptom, it was described as upper lumbar in 22 per cent, lower thoracic in 6 per cent, lower thoracic and entire lumbar in 3 per cent and lumbosacral in 1 per cent (Table 4–3).

On the initial physical examination jaundice was noted in 40 per cent of patients, an enlarged liver in 19 per cent and a palpable

*TABLE 4-3.   PANCREATIC ADENOCARCINOMA (239 PATIENTS):
FREQUENCY AND ORDER OF APPEARANCE OF BACK PAIN**

			PATIENTS WITH PAIN AT SITE			
			Order of Appearance of Pain			
SITE OF PAIN	No.	*% of* 239	*1*	*2*	*3*	*4*
			Patients			
Lower thoracic	32	13	14 (6)†	10	8	0
Upper lumbar	90	38	52 (22)	28	10	0
Lower thoracic and entire lumbar	11	5	6 (3)	2	2	1
Lumbosacral	6	3	2 (1)	4	0	0

*From Gambill, E. E.: Pancreatic and ampullary carcinoma: Diagnosis and prognosis in relationship to symptoms, physical findings, and elapse of time as observed in 255 patients. South. Med. J. 63:1120, 1970. Reprinted by permission from The Southern Medical Journal.

†Number in parentheses is percent of 239 patients.

gallbladder in 12 per cent. Other less common physical findings included fever in 9 per cent, thrombophlebitis in 3 per cent, splenomegaly in 2 per cent and ascites in 2 per cent.

The significance of these symptom complexes is illustrated by the observation that the greatest delay in diagnosis occurred when the symptoms were abdominal pain, epigastric bloating, vomiting and upper gastrointestinal bleeding, whereas the diagnosis was made with the shortest delay when the symptoms included anorexia, nausea, dark-colored urine, pruritus, weight loss, constipation and chills. The mean duration of the interval from the onset of symptoms to diagnosis was 4 months.

Another, more recent retrospective review of 100 patients with pancreatic carcinoma concluded that 36 per cent of patients reported weight loss, 32 per cent abdominal pain, 25 per cent jaundice, 32 per cent anorexia and 26 per cent nausea. The average interval between the onset of symptoms and admission to the hospital was 3 months. On physical examination, jaundice was noted in 58 per cent, an abdominal mass in 24 per cent and hepatomegaly in 40 per cent. The gallbladder was palpable in 7 per cent, and splenomegaly was noted in only 1 per cent.[88]

Until recently classification of the location of pancreatic cancer into the head, body or tail of the pancreas was possible only in surgical or autopsy cases. In one representative series, the tumor was in the head in 60 per cent, in the head and body in 5 per cent, in the body in 14 per cent, in the body and tail in 10 per cent and in the tail in 2 per cent, with nine patients omitted from the classification.[43] In another series of 236 patients operated upon from 1932 to 1962, the tumor was in the head in 126, in the body in 101 and in the tail in 9.[36] Between 1943 and 1970 at Charity Hospital in New Orleans, 449 patients were seen with histologically proven malignant tumors of the pancreas. The head was the main site in 306 patients, the body in 64 and the tail in 50. The tumor involved the pancreas diffusely in 29 patients.[40] Tables 4–4 and 4–5 show the symptoms and signs recorded in patients with cancer of the pancreas according to the location of the tumor. Note that cancer of the head of the pancreas was characterized by relatively less abdominal pain but a high percentage of the patients had jaundice, whereas in patients with cancer of the body, abdominal pain was present in 96 per cent and jaundice in only 13.6 per cent, but back pain was present in nearly twice as great a percentage as in patients with cancer of the head. The symptoms of patients with cancer of the tail of the pancreas resembled those of patients with cancer of the body. In this series the initial symptoms were related to metastatic tumor in 1.6 per cent of patients with cancer of the head but in 21.7 per cent of those with cancer of the body (Table 4–4).

In another large series of patients who were operated on, 62 per cent of those with carcinoma of the head had pain. Of these, only 8 were not jaundiced, whereas among the patients with cancer of the

TABLE 4–4. SYMPTOMS*

	NUMBER OF PATIENTS			
	63	22	7	91
		Body	Unclas-	
	Head	and Tail	sified	Total
SYMPTOMS		% Incidence		
Weight loss	85.5	86.4	85.7	85.7
Abdominal pain	76.2	96.0	85.7	83.5
Anorexia	72.6	72.7	71.4	72.6
Jaundice	71.0	13.6	30.0	53.8
Constipation	40.3	72.7	51.4	49.4
Nausea	40.3	41.0	42.9	40.7
Weakness and fatigue	41.9	45.4	14.3	40.7
Gas	32.3	18.2	30.0	28.6
Vomiting	29.0	22.7	14.3	26.3
Diarrhea	19.4	18.2	14.3	18.7
Indigestion	19.4	13.6	14.3	17.6
Fullness after eating	17.7	9.1	14.3	15.4
Back pain	13.0	22.7	14.3	15.4
Edema	6.3	27.3	25.0	13.2
Hematemesis	4.8	4.5	0	4.4
Fatty food intolerance	6.5	0	0	4.4
Initial symptoms from metastases	1.6	21.7	12.5	7.7

*From Gullick, H. D.: Carcinoma of the pancreas: A review and critical study of 100 cases. Medicine 38:48, 1959. © 1959 The Williams & Wilkins Co., Baltimore.

TABLE 4–5. PHYSICAL EXAMINATION*

	NUMBER OF PATIENTS			
	65	25	8	97
		Body	Unclas-	
	Head	and Tail	sified	Total
PHYSICAL SIGNS		% Incidence		
Jaundice	89.1	28.0	25.0	68.0
Palpable liver	68.9	44.0	88.0	64.0
Abdominal tenderness	49.0	52.0	62.5	61.0
Palpable gallbladder	37.5	4.0	12.5	26.8
Abdominal mass	15.6	36.0	50.0	23.7
Ascites	20.3	36.0	0	22.7
Edema	17.1	36.0	25.0	22.7
Palpable spleen	4.6	0	0	3.1

*From Gullick, H. D.: Carcinoma of the pancreas: A review and critical study of 100 cases. Medicine 38:57, 1959. © 1959 The Williams & Wilkins Co., Baltimore.

body, 91 per cent complained of pain but only 13 of 101 were jaundiced. Diabetes of recent origin was present in 9 of 126 patients with cancer of the head, thrombophlebitis in 5 and diarrhea in 14. Only 2 of these patients gave a history suggesting steatorrhea. Of the patients with cancer of the body, 73 per cent reported weight loss, 6 per cent had diabetes, 3 per cent had anorexia and vomiting and 6 per cent had a massive gastrointestinal bleed. The interval between the onset of symptoms and operation was nearly twice as long for patients with cancer of the body and tail as for those with cancer of the head.[36]

The clinical syndromes presenting in patients with carcinoma of the pancreas include the following: (1) obstructive jaundice; (2) metastatic malignant disease with the primary site unknown; (3) malabsorption syndrome; (4) acute cholecystitis; (5) acute pancreatitis; (6) peptic ulcer syndrome; (7) mental depression; (8) back pain; (9) thromboembolism; (10) pulmonary metastases; (11) diabetes; and (12) polyarthritis and skin nodules.

Some of the symptoms and signs require further comment. An important factor in the palpation of an enlarged gallbladder is the degree of relaxation of the abdominal wall. Having the patient bend at the knees will help, and if the examiner has warm hands it will be easier. It is good practice to return on several occasions to palpate the abdomen if relaxation is hard to obtain. Even with all these precautions, the gallbladder will be found to be enlarged and palpable in a higher percentage of patients on the operating table after the administration of anesthesia than before.

The prominence of neuropsychiatric symptoms as features of patients with carcinoma of the pancreas is of interest. In a consecutive series of 46 patients from the Mayo Clinic, 76 per cent had psychiatric symptoms related to pancreatic cancer, and in nearly half of them, the psychiatric symptoms appeared before any others.[31] Depression was the most common clinical feature. Loss of ambition was also a common complaint. That these features are more common in patients with pancreatic cancer is suggested by the fact that in another series at the same clinic only 17 per cent of patients with carcinoma of the colon had similar symptoms.

Multiple skin nodules representing fat necrosis can be a dramatic feature of pancreatic cancer.[26] The nodules are elevated, red and tender and suggest cellulitis. Most patients with nodules already have metastases.[39] The Weber-Christian syndrome of nodular panniculitis has been found to be due to cancer of the pancreas in 25 patients reported in the literature.[17] Eosinophilia was present in 14 of the patients.

Pancreatic carcinoma is one of the most common malignant tumors associated with the production of hormones by cells of the tumor. Cushing's syndrome due to production of an ACTH-like peptide is an example.[44] Some tumors have produced melanocyte-stimulating hormone as well. Gonadotropins also have been produced by pancreatic tumors, with corresponding effects on the reproductive organs.[80]

Rarely, patients with pancreatic cancer present with symptoms and signs of acute pancreatitis, including pseudocysts and abscesses. This may occur in the last trimester of pregnancy.[10] A stone in the pancreatic duct associated with pancreatitis and pancreatic carcinoma has been reported.[69]

A hemolytic anemia with severe jaundice may complicate pancreatic cancer and account for serum bilirubin levels above 30 mg/100 ml.[16]

These descriptions of the presentation of patients with pancreatic carcinoma have emphasized the broad spectrum of the disease. In terms of the resectability of the tumor, it must be admitted that there are few early symptoms; pain, abdominal fullness, nausea and vomiting, loss of appetite, weight loss and jaundice (in cancer of the head of the pancreas) probably represent the earliest symptoms and signs.

RISK FACTORS IN THE DIAGNOSIS OF PANCREATIC CARCINOMA

In order to identify patients with a high risk of developing pancreatic cancer and hence to sharpen the physician's diagnostic acumen, it is worthwhile to consider what is currently known about risk factors. A history of prolonged periods of occupational exposure to chemical and industrial toxins may be important. Studies of members of the American Chemical Society indicated a higher than normal risk of pancreatic cancer.[62]

Cigarette smoking is more common in patients with pancreatic cancer than in the general population, and smokers of more than 10 to 20 cigarettes a day may have an increased risk, about twice that of nonsmokers.[50, 53] Diabetics appear to have a greater risk of developing pancreatic cancer. From 5 to 60 per cent of all malignant tumors in patients with diabetes may be pancreatic cancers.[12] This may reach two to eight times the risk of pancreatic cancer in the general population in women.[89] The relation of chronic pancreatitis to pancreatic cancer is controversial. About 10 per cent of patients with carcinoma of the pancreas have a significant degree of histopathologic pancreatitis, but the syndrome of acute pancreatitis is rare in the course of pancreatic cancer.[4] About 1 per cent of patients with cancer of the pancreas have calcifications in the pancreas, but the percentage of patients with pancreatic calcification who have pancreatic cancer is higher.[65, 70] Interestingly, alcohol abuse does not appear to be a significant risk factor for pancreatic cancer.[57] Therefore, particular attention should be paid to the possibility of pancreatic cancer in patients with prolonged exposure to industrial toxins, long history of tobacco abuse, diabetes mellitus and chronic pancreatitis or pancreatic calcification.

LABORATORY DIAGNOSIS OF PANCREATIC CARCINOMA

A conclusive diagnosis of carcinoma of the pancreas can be established only by cytologic examination or biopsy. Earlier studies by expert cytologists indicated that in about half the patients with pancreatic cancer duodenal fluid obtained with a single-lumen tube would show class 4 or 5 cytologic findings.[66] Double-lumen intubation of the stomach and duodenum and stimulation with secretin CCK did not improve the results significantly. The results of cytologic examination of specimens obtained by passing a brush through the cannula during retrograde endoscopic pancreatography are not significantly better, but the material was said to be richer in tumor cells and to contain better preserved cells.[68]

An encouraging preliminary account of cytologic study of material obtained from the pancreatic duct by aspiration at ERCP during secretin stimulation reported that a diagnosis of cancer was made in 11 of 14 patients but, more significantly, that 13 of the patients underwent resection and 4 survived more than 1 year.[27]

For many years biopsy of the pancreas for the histologic diagnosis of pancreatic carcinoma was regarded as dangerous because of the risk of producing a pancreatic fistula. More recently, aspiration biopsy of the pancreas with a small-gauge needle at the time of laparotomy has been found to carry little risk of fistula and to result in cytologic evidence of malignancy in a high percentage of cases, e.g., 18 of 21,[77] 21 of 25 patients,[30] and 27 of 45 patients with a palpable mass in the pancreas. In the last series, the remaining 18 patients included 10 with chronic pancreatitis and 8 with penetrating ulcers. There was one false-positive result among 37 patients.[32] Some surgeons still prefer a wedge biopsy to a needle biopsy in all but periampullary lesions, citing evidence that only 5 per cent had complications, but a Vim-Silverman needle was used in the needle biopsies.[55] Failures of biopsy have uniformly been false negatives. Percutaneous needle biopsy of pancreatic masses has also been introduced for the diagnosis of pancreatic carcinoma. Guidance of the needle can be obtained with the use of ultrasonography,[29, 37, 79] computerized axial tomography (CAT scan)[28] or fluoroscopy.[38] The numbers of patients are small but the positive results are encouraging in terms of saving of costs of procedures and hospitalization.[41] Representative results are positive biopsies in 19 of 31 patients,[38] 6 of 11,[37] 5 of 7[79] and 9 of 12.[28] In patients with locally unresectable lesions, as judged by angiography, liver scan or previous laparotomy, aspiration biopsy showed tumor cells in 24 of 31 patients.[71] Fine-needle aspiration biopsy of the pancreas can be performed during retrograde cannulation of the pancreatic duct through the fiberoptic endoscope.[47] Aspiration biopsy can also be performed by a transduodenal or transgastric route through a side-viewing fiberoptic duodenoscope. This procedure yielded a positive diagnosis in 10 of 12 patients.[86]

All other methods of diagnosis of pancreatic carcinoma are indirect. Routine blood and urine determinations are helpful in detecting anemia and jaundice, particularly in patients who might otherwise be treated for functional gastrointestinal disease. Elevations of the serum bilirubin or blood sugar may be supportive of the diagnosis of pancreatic disease. Elevations can be expected in about 40 per cent of patients.[88] Abnormal glucose tolerance will be found in about 70 per cent of patients with pancreatic carcinoma, particularly late in the disease. Elevations of alkaline phosphatase occur in about 40 per cent of patients and support the diagnosis of obstructive jaundice. The significance can be confirmed with the serum 5' nucleotidase to differentiate sources of alkaline phosphatase from bone. On the other hand, neither the serum nor urine amylase level has been very helpful in the diagnosis of pancreatic cancer.[35] Low levels of pancreatic isoamylase can be found in patients with pancreatic cancer or chronic pancreatitis with normal total serum amylases, but this technique is still not available as a routine laboratory procedure.[78] The serum AIT (SGOT) is modestly elevated in 80 per cent of patients, but a positive test for occult blood in the stool has been reported in more than half the patients.[88]

Carcinoma of the pancreas is associated with elevations in the serum levels of carcinoembryonic antigen above 2.5 mg/ml in a majority of patients.[67] Higher levels were associated with metastases and shorter survival.[56] Elevations of CEA also occur in patients with chronic pancreatitis, however.[18, 19] In both pancreatic cancer and chronic pancreatitis higher levels of CEA are present in the pancreatic juice than in the serum or plasma.[75] These results so far have indicated that CEA levels are unlikely to be useful in the early detection of pancreatic cancer.

Detection of impaired secretory capacity of the pancreas in patients with pancreatic cancer is of value primarily in those patients in whom pancreatic disease is not clinically evident and it would be helpful to know whether the patient has *pancreatic* disease, rather than whether the specific disease is cancer. In the largest series reported, 231 of 242 patients with cancer of the head of the pancreas had abnormal responses in volume, bicarbonate concentration or bicarbonate output to intravenous administration of secretin; abnormal responses were found in somewhat fewer patients with carcinoma of the body or tail of the pancreas (80 to 83 per cent).[25] There is no evidence that use of a maximally stimulating dose of secretin would improve these results. The impression that a low volume response as compared to a low bicarbonate concentration would reliably differentiate pancreatic cancer from chronic pancreatitis has not been confirmed.

Routine radiologic examinations such as barium meals and barium enemas can provide only evidence of encroachment of pancreatic cancers on the lumen of the gastrointestinal tract (Table 4–6). They may provide clues in patients in whom the diagnosis has not previously been suspected but are unlikely help in the diagnosis of early and curable disease. Ulcerating lesions of the postbulbar duodenum may prove to be due to pancreatic carcinoma.[7] Hypotonic duodenography in which the musculature of the duodenum is relaxed by agents such as the anticholinergic drug propantheline or the hormone glucagon permits better visualization of the duodenum for detection of encroachment by pancreatic tumors, but again this is a late manifestation, and there is currently little enthusiasm for the procedure.[3] Pancreatic scintiscanning with selenomethionine has not been very helpful.

Percutaneous transhepatic cholangiography with the "skinny" needle has proved to be a valuable diagnostic aid in patients with pancreatic carcinoma and jaundice.[49] The ducts can be visualized in most patients, e.g., 29 of 33 patients with pancreatic cancer, but failure of visualization may result in false-negative reports.[49] The nature of the filling defect at the lower end of the common duct is not always sufficiently diagnostic to distinguish between cancer and common duct stone. Rare examples of patients with both diseases have been observed.

Endoscopic retrograde cholangiopancreatography (ERCP) by means of injecting a radiopaque medium into the pancreatic duct after cannulation under direct vision using a side-viewing fiberoptic duodenoscope permits the detection of obstruction or filling defects within the pancreatic ducts. Main duct occlusion with a regular reduction in caliber was found in 14 of 25 patients with pancreatic cancer but in only 5 of 24 patients with chronic pancreatitis.[51] Normal

*TABLE 4–6.   ROENTGENOLOGIC EXAMINATIONS**

	G.I. Series		Barium Enema		Cholecystogram	
		%		%		%
	No. of	Positive	No. of	Positive	No. of	Positive
SITE OF TUMOR	Patients	Findings	Patients	Findings	Patients	Findings
Head	36	52.8	9	11.0	17	64.7
Body and tail	18	44.4	7	29.0	7	14.3
Unclassified	6	50.0	4	25.0	2	0
Total	60	50.0	20	20.0	26	46.2

*From Gullick, H. D.: Carcinoma of the pancreas: A review and critical study of 100 cases. Medicine 38:65, 1959. © 1959 The Williams & Wilkins Co., Baltimore.

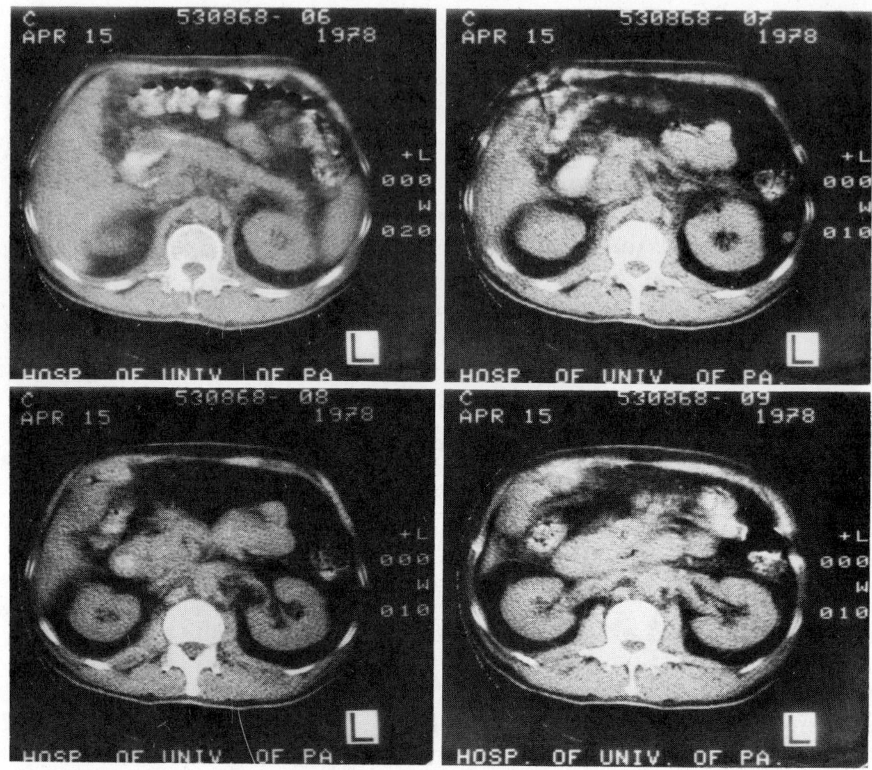

Figure 4–1.   Computerized axial tomography (CAT) scan from a patient with carcinoma of the pancreas. There is a small mass involving the head of the pancreas. (Courtesy of Dr. Herbert Y. Kressel, Department of Radiology, Hospital of the University of Pennsylvania.)

ducts were reported in 20 per cent of patients with pancreatic cancer.[13] On the other hand, occlusion of the ducts was irregular in 14 and the caliber was variable in 20 of the patients with pancreatitis but in only 5 and 4, respectively, of the patients with carcinoma. ERCP was more accurate than a secretin-CCK test in the diagnosis of pancreatic cancer.[74] Carcinoma of the ampulla of Vater can be seen and biopsied under direct vision during ERCP.

Much current interest centers on the possible value of ultrasonography and CAT scanning in the diagnosis of pancreatic carcinoma. Ultrasonography is relatively inexpensive and does not expose the patient to ionizing radiation. Abnormal dimensions of the pancreas have been recognized in patients with pancreatic cancer, but the finding is not specific for cancer.[29, 52, 59] No evidence of longer survival was noted among patients whose carcinoma was detected by ultrasonography.[2] CAT scans also detect abnormalities in the dimensions of the pancreas but currently are expensive and expose the patient to ionizing radiation (Fig. 4–1). It is not yet known whether CAT scans offer sufficient advantage over ultrasonography to justify the additional costs and hazards.[63] Pseudocysts may coexist with carcinoma of the pancreas.

Selective arteriography has enjoyed considerable popularity in the United States for the diagnosis of pancreatic carcinoma. Encasement of the vessels by tumor is the most reliable criterion for diagnosis.[64] Abnormal vessels are the next most common abnormality.[8] Mild compression to complete occlusion of the splenic vein as seen during the venous phase of angiography is an important sign, especially in carcinoma of the body and tail of the pancreas.[11] Some correlation between the extent of the tumor as detected on angiography and the patient's survival has been noted.[82, 87] Encasement of the gastroduodenal artery but not of the large extrapancreatic arteries was found in 26 patients, and of whom 6 had a resectable tumor and a longer survival time.[87] Current opinion minimizes the value of angiography in the diagnosis of pancreatic carcinoma except in cystadenocarcinoma or islet cell tumor, in which the tumor blush may be characteristic.[3a]

Reports from clinical units where laparoscopy is practiced indicate that it is of value in detecting metastases, performing cholangiography and performing biopsy of suspected tumors of the pancreas.[15]

Laparotomy is still often the final diagnostic study for the diagnosis of pancreatic carcinoma. Unfortunately, it may not be possible to differentiate between cancer and chronic pancreatitis by inspection and palpation in the absence of metastases, and biopsy of a lymph node does not reveal the primary site even when tumor is present.

Because of the limitations of the various diagnostic methods, attention has been directed to combinations of diagnostic procedures. Given the current concern about medical costs, it is of great importance to choose the least costly but most effective diagnostic procedures. Combinations of secretin tests, duodenal cytologic study and hypotonic duodenography;[9] selective arteriography and hypotonic duodenography;[83] and percutaneous transhepatic cholangiography, hypotonic duodenography and cytologic study[84] have been tested without clear evidence that any of the combinations shortens the time to diagnosis, reduces the cost or improves the survival. Comparisons of serum CEA determinations with the CCK test for duodenal enzymes showed the latter to be more reliable.[21] CAT scans were superior to ultrasonography in one study of 33 patients with carcinoma of the pancreas,[2] but none of the patients had resectable lesions. ERCP was superior to CAT scans and ultrasonography in patients with pancreatic cancer presenting with pain but equivalent to them in patients with a pancreatic mass.[14] CAT scans were judged superior to ultrasonography. A prospective evaluation of 70 patients with pancreatic carcinoma at the Mayo Clinic included CCK stimulation of duodenal enzymes, pancreatic scans, thermography, ultrasonography and ERCP. The results led the authors to recommend the following algorithm: ultrasonography as the first study; if negative, followed by CCK stimulation; if positive, followed by ERCP.[22] This protocol would permit identification of 89 per cent of patients with pancreatic cancer.

It is obvious that a diagnostic algorithm that could permit identification of pancreatic carcinoma at an early stage when surgery might be curative, and at the same time reduce the preoperative period of hospitalization and avoid laboratory tests that contribute little to the diagnosis, would be a very useful guide to the physician responsible for the study of patients suspected of having pancreatic cancer. This is not possible at present for two reasons: no single laboratory diagnostic procedure or combination of procedures has been shown to permit identification of resectable cancers of the pancreas, and there are as yet no conclusive data to establish the superiority of any individual procedure in the diagnosis of pancreatic cancer at any stage.[20, 33]

In the meantime, physicians must make reasonable and prudent choices in patients requiring study. Ultrasonography and CAT scans have the greater appeal of being well tolerated, noninvasive procedures. It is not yet known with certainty what the minimal size of a pancreatic tumor is that can be detected by these techniques. Ultrasonography requires a well trained person for the interpretation of the sonographs. It has the advantages of being relatively less expensive than CAT scans and free of the danger of ionizing radiation. CAT scans are superb examples of cross-sectional gross anatomy, which are readily appreciated by most physicians. They do expose the patient to radiation, and they are very expensive. While awaiting the information noted above, it seems reasonable to include one or the other of these examinations in the early phase of laboratory studies of patients suspected of having pancreatic cancer. In the jaundiced patient, the next step may well be percutaneous transhepatic cholangiography if blood coagulation is normal or ERCP if a competent endoscopist is available. In patients without jaundice, collection of duodenal content during stimulation of the pancreas with secretin and CCK is probably the most sensitive test for abnormalities in pancreatic function. If a pancreatic mass lesion can be identified, percutaneous needle biopsy of the mass under guidance of ultrasonography or CAT scan may be the most direct approach to the diagnosis short of laparotomy. Angiography seems to be of some value in determining resectability, but this requires further study in a controlled design.

DIAGNOSIS AND DIFFERENTIAL DIAGNOSIS OF PANCREATIC CARCINOMA

It must be said that there are at present no recognized symptoms or signs of early pancreatic cancer. The laboratory diagnostic studies that are available for the study of patients with suspected pancreatic cancer are among the more costly in gastroenterology and there is at present no assurance that their routine use will improve the survival rate in this grim disease. The physician is caught in the dilemma of whether to accept minimal clinical evidence from the history and physical examination as an indication for a full investigation leading to surgical exploration or to wait until more definite indications are present and face the likelihood that the diagnosis will be made too late to offer the patient anything put palliation.[20] In this situation the primary care physician who has followed the patient for years has a advantage in detecting subtle changes over long periods of time. On the other hand, this situation can also delay the diagnosis if the patient has been treated for functional bowel disturbances and the physician does not make periodic re-evaluations of the patients' symptoms and signs. The conscientious consultant may feel obligated to pursue the diagnosis to a definite conclusion once the patient has been referred by a competent primary care physician.

The major indication for a provisional diagnosis of cancer of the pancreas is persistent upper abdominal distress that has none of the characteristics of that of other types of intra-abdominal disease, e.g., relieved by food or a bowel movement, associated with emotional stress, or following an intermittent pattern. Significant weight loss and resort to analgesics for pain relief are cues that should raise the index of suspicion. In cancer of the head of the pancreas, generalized itching and dark urine precede the recognition of jaundice. In cancer of the body and tail, pain may be referred to the back, and the chances are greater that the patient will present with a malabsorption syndrome.

The differential diagnosis of pancreatic cancer includes other causes of obstructive jaundice in the case of cancer of the head of the pancreas, mental depression and symptoms of the irritable bowel syndrome, malabsorption syndrome due to maldigestion and obscure causes of abdominal and back pain in cancer of the body and tail. Probably the most challenging differential diagnosis is between early pancreatic carcinoma and chronic pancreatitis. In some patients the clinical syndrome is dominated by metastatic lesions, such as multiple metastatic lesions in the lung or liver metastases with hepatomegaly, and the differential diagnosis must include other primary tumors or other causes of hepatomegaly. Secondary metastatic cancer to the pancreas is rare.[54]

THE COURSE OF PANCREATIC CARCINOMA

Unfortunately the inexorable course of this dreadful disease is well known. About one third of patients live less than a month after the diagnosis is established, another third live 1 to 3 months, about 15 per cent live 3 to 6 months and another 15 per cent survive more than 6 months.[36] In a study in Minnesota, 11 per cent survived 1 year. All

*TABLE 4–7.   SITES OF METASTASES AT AUTOPSY**

	Number of Autopsies				
	49	19	1	69	TOTAL
		Body	Unclas-		NUMBER
SITE OF	Head	and Tail	sified	Total	OF
METASTASIS		% Incidence			PATIENTS
Liver	57.3	63.2	0	59.6	40
Regional nodes	57.3	42.1	100	53.6	37
Peritoneum	30.6	68.4	0	40.6	28
Lung	24.5	31.6	100	27.5	19
G-I tract	4.1	26.3	0	10.1	7
Diaphragm, adrenal gland	4.1	21.1	0	8.7	6
Kidney	0	15.8	0	4.3	3
Mediastinal nodes	2.0	5.3	100	4.3	3
Pericardium	4.1	5.3	0	4.3	3
Pleura	2.0	10.5	0	4.3	3
Cervical nodes	2.0	5.3	0	2.9	2
Bone marrow	2.0	5.3	0	2.9	2
Vertebrae, spleen	0	10.5	0	2.9	2
Rib, uterus	2.0	0	0	1.5	1
Bronchial nodes Esophageal nodes Axillary nodes Retrobulbar fat Epidural space Spermatic cord Psoas muscle Ureter, ovary Tubes, cervix Vagina	0	5.3	0	1.5	1

*From Gullick, H. D.: Carcinoma of the pancreas: A review and critical study of 100 cases. Medicine 38:72, 1959. © 1959 The Williams & Wilkins Co., Baltimore.

the patients were dead within 3 years. A staging protocol developed by the American Cancer Society indicates that survival can be clearly linked to the extent of the disease and to the course of the patient after surgical procedures. Table 4–7 shows the distribution of metastases at autopsy in patients with carcinoma of the pancreas.[43] It can be seen that metastases to the liver developed in 60 per cent of patients and metastases to the regional lymph nodes in almost as many. Peritoneal metastases were present in 40 per cent and lung metastases in about 25 per cent. The usual cause of failure of radical surgical resection is local recurrence, which may appear years later.[76]

The most difficult problem in patients with pancreatic cancer is usually persistent abdominal pain, but in some patients nausea and vomiting or pruritus may be dominant features.

Prognostic factors for resectability of pancreatic carcinoma include a lesion less than 9 sq cm in size, the absence of pain, the presence of jaundice and location of the lesion in the head of the pancreas.[1]

TREATMENT OF PANCREATIC CARCINOMA

We have just passed through a phase of profound therapeutic nihilism in the management of patients with pancreatic cancer. The Whipple procedure — removal of the duodenum and proximal two thirds of the pancreas — fell into disrepute because of the mortality and short survival time. Now total pancreatectomy is being considered as an alternative, and more emphasis is being placed on the selection for these procedures of patients in whom the mortality and morbidity will be reasonably low and in whom long survivals can be achieved. It remains to be seen what the outcome of such surgical procedures will be, but at present, considering the otherwise predictably fatal course of the disease, it seems reasonable to inform patients with favorable characteristics of the possibility of surgical benefit and to permit them to participate in the decision whether to attempt a surgical cure.[85a] In a group of 393 patients, the average survival of patients with a lesion less than 30 sq cm was 41 weeks, compared to 22 weeks for those with large lesions. In jaundiced patients a biliary bypass operation was associated with a 36-week survival, compared to 19 weeks for those without a bypass. The influence of factors determining the choice of procedure is unknown.[1] Some radiotherapists have reported significant improvement in survival of patients with cancer of the pancreas following cobalt therapy, and subsequent studies need to be evaluated carefully.[45] Chemotherapy has been disappointing, but new protocols continue to be developed and tested. Since weight loss in pancreatic carcinoma is best related to malabsorption, it is important to note that supplemental pancreatic extracts can correct the malabsorption. Incidentally, the triolein breath test identified the six of nine patients with moderate to severe fat malabsorption in whom the fat malabsorption was best corrected by pancreatic extracts. Fat malabsorption was less but not totally corrected, while protein malabsorption was totally corrected in three of five patients.[72]

EPIDEMIOLOGY OF PANCREATIC CARCINOMA

The incidence of pancreatic carcinoma in the United States has increased in the last two decades, especially among nonwhite males.[50, 53] It is now the fourth leading cause of death among cancer of all sites (Fig. 4–2). There has been no improvement in survival over three decades. There is an interesting relationship between pancreatic and gastric cancer. In general, the incidence is inversely related. In the United States, the decrease in incidence of gastric cancer has been matched by a rise in incidence of pancreatic cancer.[81] A similar phenomenon has been noted in other countries. Recently, cancer of the pancreas in Olmstead County, Minnesota, from 1935 to 1974 has

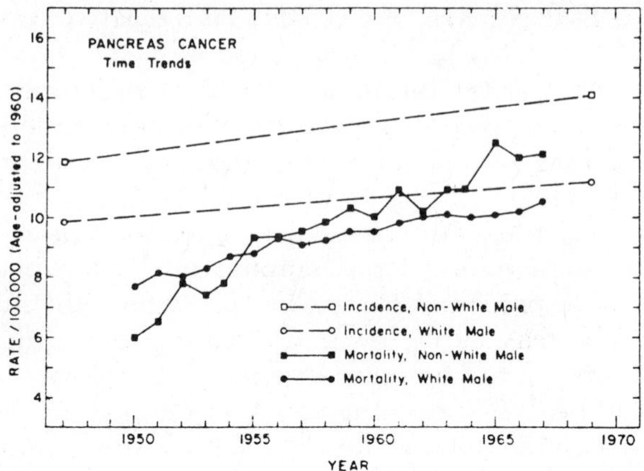

Figure 4–2. Trends in the incidence of carcinoma of the pancreas in the United States over 20 years. (From Levine, D. L., and Connelly, R. R.: Cancer of the pancreas. Available epidemiologic information and its implications. Cancer 31:1232, 1973.)

been reviewed.[58] The annual incidence rate was 7.4 per 100,000 for men and 3.5 per 100,000 for women. Almost 75 per cent of the patients were over 65 years of age.

PATHOPHYSIOLOGY OF PANCREATIC CARCINOMA

The pathophysiology is essentially that of obstructive jaundice and malabsorption due to loss of pancreatic enzymes when the pancreatic duct becomes obstructed. It should be remembered that the absence of bile from the alimentary canal reduces the absorption of fat-soluble vitamins, particularly vitamin K. Bulky pancreatic tumors can obstruct the outlet of the stomach by extrinsic pressure or actually invade the duodenum or jejunum at the ligament of Treitz or the transverse colon. Invasion of the splenic vein may cause gastric varices and lead to gastrointestinal bleeding. Only 1 per cent of all pancreatic adenocarcinomas produce digestive enzymes.[89]

Evidence from balance studies indicates that weight loss in pancreatic carcinoma correlates better with the extent of malabsorption of fat and protein than with the amount of calories uneaten on a standard diet.[73]

Histologic examination of the pancreaticoduodenal area after block removal at 353 postmortem examinations showed that the absence of a well developed common pancreaticobiliary channel at the entrance to the duodenum was associated with epithelial abnormalities, including papillary hyperplasia, of the main pancreatic duct in 30 per cent of patients, compared to 19 per cent of patients with a well developed common channel.[23] These abnormalities may represent precancerous changes and hence indicate that lack of a common channel is a factor in pancreatic carcinogenesis.

ANIMAL MODELS OF PANCREATIC CARCINOMA

Models of pancreatic carcinoma in animals are now beginning to be produced by means of chemical carcinogens that are selectively taken up by pancreatic ductal cells.[5, 6] A single injection of a nitrosamine compound in hamsters can increase pancreatic protein concentration and output for at least 4 weeks. Electrolytes in pancreatic secretion were unaffected. Structural changes occur after a single injection, and carcinomas appear after 20 weeks of weekly injections. These results suggest that this carcinogen has a selective action on protein-secreting cells.[24] Perhaps the most exciting development has been a preliminary report that CCK over long periods of time may produce pancreatic carcinoma in animals.[88a] These results suggest that environmental carcinogens must be considered in the etiology of pancreatic cancer in the studies now being conducted by the Environmental Protection Agency and occupational safety authorities.

ETIOLOGY OF PANCREATIC CARCINOMA

The etiology of pancreatic cancer is unknown. It is one of the cancers of the digestive system in which familial groupings occur with an awesome frequency.[60] Most carcinomas of the pancreas arise from ductal cells, but acinar cell carcinoma and pleomorphic cell carcinomas do occur.[42] The fact that occult pancreatic carcinoma has been reported in an immunosuppressed patient indicates that this tumor may be one of those found in association with inadequate host recognition and response.[85]

SCREENING FOR PANCREATIC CARCINOMA

Development of screening procedures awaits more sensitive diagnostic methods and the identification of a population at high risk for developing pancreatic carcinoma. If a pilot study is carried out with ultrasonography for the detection of gallstones it will be interesting to see if any pancreatic carcinomas are detected.

PREVENTION OF PANCREATIC CARCINOMA

The prevention of pancreatic carcinoma is at present beyond our ability in most cases. If cigarette smokers do carry a twofold to threefold greater risk of pancreatic carcinoma, then prevention might be one more benefit of the anti-smoking campaign.[89] It is not known whether or not the risk of pancreatic carcinoma in patients with diabetes is influenced by control of the diabetes. In a recent study, statistical significance of a correlation was lost if only patients who had had diabetes for 2 years were considered.[58]

PANCREATIC CYSTADENOMA AND CYSTADENOCARCINOMA

The two reasons for identifying this rather small group of pancreatic tumors are their unusual diagnostic features and the better survival following surgical procedures than with adenocarcinoma of the pancreas. There are no characteristic features in the history of these patients except that a palpable abdominal mass may be the first sign of the tumor. Cystadenomas may be so vascular that the mass can be felt to pulsate.[3a] Among 21 patients with cystadenocarcinomas, 17 complained of abdominal pain and 9 of weight loss, and 6 were jaundiced.[46] The mean age of the patient was 61 years. Twelve patients had a palpable abdominal mass. Cystadenocarcinomas occur about half as frequently as cystadenomas. Angiography can yield dramatic findings in cystadenomas because the increased vascularity of the tumor produces a tumor blush.[3a] In cystadenocarcinoma, calcification within the substance of the pancreas may take the appearance of a sunburst.[48] On ERCP in patients with mucus-producing tumors, bubble-like filling defects within the common bile duct have been noted.[48]

Cystadenomas should be curable by surgery. Four of seven patients with cystadenocarcinoma survived at least 5 years after complete removal, and 14 per cent of patients survived 5 years after partial removal. These results show that identification of these tumors can be a rewarding exercise for the patient and physician.

REFERENCES

1. Barkin, J. S., MacIntyre, J., and Kalser, M. H.: Prognostic factors in pancreatic carcinoma. Gastroenterology 76:1094, 1979
2. Barkin, J., Vining, D., Miale, A., Gottlieb, S., Redlhammer, D. E., and Kalser, M. H.: Computerized tomography, diagnostic ultrasound and radionuclide scanning: Comparison of efficacy in diagnosis of pancreatic carcinoma. J.A.M.A. 238:2040–2042, 1977
3. Baum, M., and Howe, C. T.: Hypotonic duodenography in the diagnosis of carcinoma of the pancreas and its further use when combined with percutaneous cholangiography and pancreatic scintiscanning. Am. J. Surg. 115:519–525, 1968
3a. Bieber, W. P., and Albo, R. J.: Cystadenoma of the pancreas. Its arteriographic diagnosis. Radiology 80:776–778, 1963

4. Becker, V.: Carcinoma of the pancreas and chronic pancreatitis — a possible relationship. Acta Hepatogastroenterol. 25:257–259, 1978
5. Black, O.: Histofluorescence of 3-methylcholanthrene metabolites in the rat pancreas. Gastroenterology 75:438–444, 1978
6. Black, O., Jr., and Webster, P. D., III: Uptake of methylcholanthrene in the rat pancreas. Am. J. Dig. Dis. 19:37–42, 1974
7. Blatt, C. J., Bernstein, R. G., and Lopez, F.: Uncommon roentgenologic manifestation of pancreatic carcinoma. Am. J. Roentgenol. 113:119–124, 1971
8. Bookstein, J. J., Reuter, S. R., and Martel, W.: Angiographic evaluation of pancreatic carcinoma. Radiology 93:757–764, 1969
9. Bourke, M. B., Swann, J. C., Brown, C. L., and Ritchie, H. D.: Exocrine pancreatic function studies, duodenal cytology and hypotonic duodenography in the diagnosis of surgical jaundice. Lancet 1:605–608, 1972
10. Boyle, J. M., and McLeod, M. E.: Pancreatic cancer presenting as pancreatitis of pregnancy. Am. J. Gastroenterol. 70:371–373, 1979
11. Buranasiri, S., and Baum, S.: The significance of the venous phase of celiac and superior mesenteric arteriography in evaluating pancreatic carcinoma. Radiology 102:11–20, 1972
12. Cohen, G. F.: Early diagnosis of pancreatic neoplasms in diabetics. Lancet 2:267–269, 1965
13. Cotton, P. B.: Progress report: Cannulation of the papilla of Vater by endoscopy and retrograde cholangiopancreatography. Gut 13:1014–1025, 1972
14. Cotton, P. B., Denyer, M. E., Kreel, L., Husband, J., Meire, H. B., and Lees, W.: Comparative clinical impact of endoscopic pancreatography, grey-scale ultrasonography and computed tomograph (EMI scanning) in pancreatic disease: Preliminary report. Gut 19:679–684, 1978
15. Cuschieri, A., Hall, A. W., and Clark, J.: Value of laparoscopy in the diagnosis and management of pancreatic carcinoma. Gut 19:672–677, 1978
16. Davis, L. J.: Symptomatic haemolytic anemia. A report of four cases. Edinburgh Med. J. 51:70–83, 1944
17. Delamarre, J., Capron, J-P., Chivrac, D., Dupas, J. L., Gortier, M. F., and Lorriaux, A.: Syndrome de Weber-Christian et cancer du pancréas. Etude d'un cas et revue de la littérature. Gastroenterol. Clin. Biol. 1:789–798, 1977
18. Delwiche, R., Zamcheck, N., and Marcon, N.: Carcinoembryonic antigen in pancreatitis. Cancer 31:328–330, 1973
19. Dilawari, J. B., Philippakos, D., Blendis, L. M., and Waller, S. L.: Carcinoembryonic antigen in differential diagnosis of carcinoma of pancreas from chronic pancreatitis. Br. Med. J. 2:668–669, 1975
20. DiMagno, E. P.: Pancreatic cancer: A continuing diagnostic dilemma. Ann. Intern. Med. 90:847–848, 1979
21. DiMagno, E. P., Malagelada, J. R., Moertel, C. G., and Go, V. L. W.: Prospective evaluation of the pancreatic secretion of immunoreactive carcinoembryonic antigen, enzyme and bicarbonate in patients suspected of having pancreatic cancer. Gastroenterology 73:457–461, 1977
22. DiMagno, E. P., Malagelada, J. R., Taylor, W. F., and Go, V. L. W.: A prospective comparison of current diagnostic tests for pancreatic cancer. New Eng. J. Med. 297:737–742, 1977
23. DiMagno, E. P., Shorter, R. G., Go, V. L. W., and Taylor, W. F.: Abnormal epithelium of the main pancreatic duct is related to pancreaticobiliary ductal anatomy. Gastroenterology 76:1122, 1979
24. Doria, J. C., Mosely, J. G., and Reber, H. A.: Single exposure to a carcinogen: Effect on pancreatic function. Gastroenterology 76:1124, 1979
25. Dreiling, D. A.: The early diagnosis of pancreatic cancer. Scand. J. Gastroenterol 5: Suppl. 6, pp. 115–122, 1970
26. Edelstein, J. M.: Pancreatic carcinoma with unusual metastases to the skin and subcutaneous tissues simulating cellulitis. New Eng. J. Med. 242:779–781, 1950
27. Endo, Y., Morii, T., Tamura, H., and Okuda, S.: Cytodiagnosis of pancreatic malignant tumors by aspiration under direct vision using a duodenal fiberscope. Gastroenterology 67:944–951, 1974
28. Ferrucci, J. T., Jr., and Wittenberg, J.: CT biopsy of abdominal tumors: Aids for lesion localization. Radiology 129:739–744, 1978

29. Fontana, G., Bolondi, L., Conti, M., Plicchi, G., Gullo, L., Caletti, G. C., and Labo, G.: An evaluation of echography in the diagnosis of pancreatic disease. Gut 17:228–234, 1976

30. Forsgren, L., and Orell, S.: Aspiration cytology in carcinoma of the pancreas. Surgery 73:38–42, 1973

31. Fras, I., Litin, E. M., and Pearson, J. S.: Comparison of psychiatric symptoms in carcinoma of the pancreas with those in some other intra-abdominal neoplasms. Am. J. Psychiatry 123:1553–1562, 1967

32. Frederiksen, P., Thommesen, P., and Skjoldborg, H.: Fine needle aspiration biopsy of the pancreas. Scand. J. Gastroenterol. 11:785–791, 1976

33. Freeney, P. C., and Ball, T.: Rapid diagnosis of pancreatic carcinoma: An algorithmic approach. Radiology 127:627–633, 1978

34. Gambill, E. E.: Pancreatic and ampullary carcinoma: Diagnosis and prognosis in relationship to symptoms, physicial findings, and elapse of time as observed in 255 patients. South. Med. J. 63:1119–1122, 1970

35. Gambill, E. E., and Mason, H. L.: Urinary amylase vs. serum amylase in patients with pancreatic carcinoma. J.A.M.A. 188:824–826, 1964

36. Glenn, F., and Thorbjarnarson, B.: Carcinoma of the pancreas. Ann. Surg. 159:945–958, 1964

37. Goldman, M. L., Naib, Z. M., Galambos, J. T., Rude, J. C., Kheetiang, O., Bradley, E. L., Salam, A., and Gonzalez, A. C.: Preoperative diagnosis of pancreatic carcinoma by percutaneous aspiration biopsy. Am. J. Dig. Dis. 22:1076–1082, 1977

38. Goldstein, H. M., and Zornoza, J.: Percutaneous transperitoneal aspiration biopsy of pancreatic masses. Am. J. Dig. Dis. 23:840–843, 1978

39. Good, A. E., Schnitzer, B., Kawanishi, H., Demetropoulos, K. C., and Rapp, R.: Metastatic fat necrosis: Report of a case and review of rheumatic manifestations. Am. J. Dig. Dis. 21:978–987, 1976

40. Gray, L. W., Crook, J. N., and Cohn, I.: Carcinoma of the pancreas. *In* Seventh National Cancer Conference Proceedings. Philadelphia, J. B. Lippincott Co., 1973, pp. 503–510

41. Gudjonsson, B., and Spiro, H. M.: Biopsy techniques in the diagnosis of pancreatic cancer. Gastroenterology 75:726–728, 1978

42. Guillan, R. A., and McMahon, J.: Pleomorphic adenocarcinoma of the pancreas. Am. J. Gastroenterol. 60:379–386, 1973

43. Gullick, H. D.: Carcinoma of the pancreas. A review and critical study of 100 cases. Medicine 38:47–84, 1959

44. Hallwright, G. P., North, K. A. K., and Reid, J. D.: Pigmentation and Cushing's syndrome due to malignant tumor of the pancreas. J. Clin. Endocrinol. Metab. 24:496–500, 1964

45. Haslam, J. B., Cavanaugh, P. J., and Stroup, S. L.: Radiation therapy in the treatment of irresectable adenocarcinoma of the pancreas. Cancer 32:1341–1345, 1973

46. Hodgkinson, D. J., ReMine, W. H., and Weiland, L. H.: A clinicopathologic study of 21 cases of pancreatic cystadenocarcinoma. Ann. Surg. 188:679–684, 1978

47. Ihre, T. H., Pyk, E., Raaschou-Nielsen, T., and Seligson, U.: Percutaneous fine needle aspiration biopsy during endoscopic retrograde cholangiopancreatography. Scand. J. Gastroenterol. 13:657–662, 1978

48. Ito, Y., Blackstone, M. O., Frank, P. H., and Skinner, D. B.: Mucinous biliary obstruction associated with a cystic adenocarcinoma of the pancreas. Gastroentology 73:1410–1412, 1977

49. James, M.: Normal or "negative" percutaneous cholangiography. Arch. Surg. 103:31–33, 1971

50. Krain, L. S.: The rising incidence of cancer of the pancreas — further epidemiologic studies. J. Chron. Dis. 23:685–690, 1971

51. Kruse, A., Thommesen, P., and Frederiksen, P.: Endoscopic retrograde cholangiopancreatography in pancreatic cancer and chronic pancreatitis. Differences in morphologic changes in the pancreatic duct and the bile duct. Scand. J. Gastroenterol. 13:513–518, 1978

52. Lawson, T. L.: Sensitivity of pancreatic ultrasonography in the detection of pancreatic disease. Radiology 128:733–736, 1978

53. Levine, D. L., and Connelly, R. R.: Cancer of the pancreas. Available epidemiologic information and its implications. Cancer 31:1231–1236, 1973
54. Levine, M., and Danovitch, S. H.: Metastatic carcinoma to the pancreas. Am. J. Gastroenterol. 60:290–294, 1973
55. Lightwood, R., Reber, H. A., and Way, L. W.: The risk and accuracy of pancreatic biopsy. Am. J. Surg. 132:189–194, 1976
56. Lokich, J. J., Chawla, P. L., Smith, E. H., and Zamcheck, N.: Carcinoma of the pancreas. Am. J. Gastroenterol. 62:481–487, 1974
57. Mainz, D., and Webster, P. D., III: Pancreatic carcinoma. A review of etiologic considerations. Am. J. Dig. Dis. 19:459–464, 1974
58. Maruchi, N., Brian, D., Ludwig, J., Elveback, L. R., and Kurland, L. T.: Cancer of the pancreas in Olmsted County, Minnesota, 1935–1974. Mayo Clin. Proc. 54:245–249, 1979
59. McCormack, L. R., Seat, S. G., and Strum, W. B.: Pancreatic carcinoma: Survival following detection by ultrasonic scanning. J.A.M.A. 238:240–241, 1977
60. McDermott, R. P., and Kramer, P.: Adenocarcinoma of the pancreas in four siblings. Gastroenterology 65:137–139, 1973
61. Moertel, C. G., Ahmann, D. L., Taylor, W. F., and Schwartau, N.: Aspirin and pancreatic cancer pain. Gastroenterology 60:552–553, 1971
62. Morgan, R. G. H., and Wormsley, K. G.: Cancer of the pancreas. Gut 18:580–596, 1977
63. Moss, A. A., and Kressel, H. Y.: Computed tomography of the pancreas. Am. J. Dig. Dis. 22:1018–1027, 1977
64. Ney, F. G., Feist, J. H., Altemus, L. R., and Ordinario, V. R.: The characteristic angiographic criteria of malignancy. Radiology 104:567–570, 1972
65. Noda, A., Kamiya, N., Takayama, T., and Hayakawa, T.: Pancreolithiasis and pancreatic carcinoma. Arch. Intern. Med. 137:754–760, 1977
66. Olsen, J. H.: Duodenal exfoliative cytology. Scand. J. Gastroenterol. 6:Suppl. 9, pp. 105–107, 1971
67. Ona, F. V., Zamcheck, W., Dhar, P., Moore, T., and Kupchik, H. Z.: Carcinoembryonic antigen (CEA) in the diagnosis of pancreatic cancer. Cancer 31:324–327, 1973
68. Osnes, M., Serck-Hanssen, A., and Myren, J.: Endoscopic retrograde brush cytology (ERBC) of the biliary and pancreatic ducts. Scand. J. Gastroenterol. 10:829–832, 1975
69. Parke, R., Swak, M., Cohen, M., and Talbert, W., Jr.: Pancreatitis with coexistent pancreatic duct stone and carcinoma. Arch. Intern. Med. 137:924–926, 1977
70. Paulino-Netto, A., Dreiling, D. A., and Baronofsky, I. D.: The relationship between pancreatic calcification and cancer of the pancreas. Ann. Surg. 151:530–537, 1960
71. Pereiras, R. V., Barkin, J. S., Mejen, H., Hudson, D., Levi, J., Kunhart, B., and Troner, M.: Fine needle percutaneous aspiration biopsy of pancreatic carcinoma. Gastroenterology 74:1076, 1978
72. Perez, M. M., DiMagno, E. P., Moertel, C. G., Newcomer, A. D., and Go, V. L. W.: Malabsorption is common and treatable in pancreatic cancer (PC): Predictive value of triolein breath test (TBT). Gastroenterology 76:1216, 1979
73. Perez, M. M., DiMagno, E. P., Moertel, C. G., Newcomer, A. D., and Go, V. L. W.: Why do patients with pancreatic adenocarcinoma (PC) lose weight? Gastroenterology 76:1216, 1979
74. Rolny, P., Lukes, P. J., Gamklou, R., Jagenburg, R., and Nilson, A.: A comparative evaluation of endoscopic retrograde pancreatography and secretin-CCK test in the diagnosis of pancreatic disease. Scand. J. Gastroenterol. 13:777–782, 1978
75. Sharma, M. P., Gregg, J. A., Loewenstein, M., McCabe, R. P., and Zamcheck, N.: Carcinoembryonic antigen CEA activity in pancreatic juice of patients with pancreatic carcinoma and pancreatitis. Cancer 38:2457–2461, 1976
76. Shields, H. M.: Occurrence of an adenocarcinoma at the choledochoenteric anastomosis 14 years after pancreaticoduodenectomy for benign disease. Gastroenterology 72:322–324, 1977
77. Shorey, B. A.: Aspiration biopsy of carcinoma of the pancreas. Gut 16:645–647, 1975

78. Skude, G., and Ihse, I.: Isoamylases in pancreatic carcinoma and chronic relapsing pancreatitis. Scand. J. Gastroenterol. 12:53–57, 1977
79. Smith, E. H., Bartrum, R. J., Chang, Y. C., D'Orsi, C. J., Lokich, J., Abbruzzese, A., and Dantono, J.: Percutaneous aspiration biopsy of the pancreas under ultrasonic guidance. New Eng. J. Med. 292:825–828, 1975
80. Soloway, H. B., and Sommers, S. C.: Endocrinopathy associated with pancreatic carcinomas. Ann. Surg. 164:300–304, 1966
81. Stephenson, H. E., Jr.: Cancer of the pancreas and stomach: A study in contrasts. Surgery 71:307–308, 1972
82. Suzuki, T., Kawabe, K., Imamura, M., and Honjo, I.: Survival of patients with cancer of the pancreas in relation to findings on arteriography. Ann. Surg. 176:37–41, 1972
83. Suzuki, T., Uchida, K., Kuratsuku, H., Kawabe, R., Imamura, M., and Honjo, I.: Usefulness of combined selective arteriography and hypotonic duodenography in evaluation of cancer of the pancreas. Ann. Surg. 176:791–797, 1972
84. Takeuchi, T., Kozuka, M., Ito, M., and Kato, N.: The diagnosis of cancer of the pancreas and biliary system by combined percutaneous transhepatic cholangiography, hypotonic duodenography and cytologic method. Arch. Fr. Mal. App. Dig. 61:117c, 1972
85. Tavassoli, F. A., and Lynch, R. G.: Occult adenocarcinoma of the pancreas in a 17 year old patient with immunosuppressed leukemia. Gastroenterology 66:1054–1057, 1974
85a. Tepper, J., Nardi, G., and Suit, H.: Carcinoma of the pancreas: Review of MGH Experience from 1963–1973. Cancer 37:1519–1524, 1976
86. Tsuchiya, R., Henmi, T., Kondo, N., Akashi, M., and Harada, N.: Endoscopic aspiration biopsy of the pancreas. Gastroenterology 73:1050–1052, 1977
87. Tylen, U., and Arnesjo, B.: Resectability and prognosis of carcinoma of the pancreas evaluated by angiography. Scand. J. Gastroenterol. 8:691–698, 1973
88. Weingarten, L. A., Gelb, A. M., and Fischer, M.: Pancreatic carcinoma: A clinical review and schema for evaluating patients. Presented at the American College of Gastroenterology Annual Meeting, 1978
88a. Wormsley, K. G.: In press
89. Wynder, E. L., Mabuchi, K., Maruchi, N., and Fortner, J. G.: A case control study of cancer of the pancreas. Cancer 31:641–647, 1973

CHAPTER 5

CYSTIC FIBROSIS (MUCOVISCIDOSIS)

Cystic fibrosis is the most common genetic disease of the gastrointestinal tract. It occurs in 1 of every 1500 to 4000 live births among Caucasians, and it has been estimated that the gene is carried by 1 of every 20 people in the general population.[30] Traditionally it has been considered a disease of infancy and childhood, but with improved methods of management of pulmonary infection, significant numbers of patients are surviving into adolescence and young adult life. This account will focus on these older patients, as they are most likely to be seen by the general internist.

HOW THE PATIENT WITH CYSTIC FIBROSIS PRESENTS

The predominant presenting complaints are referable to the respiratory tract, with increased sputum, cough, clubbing of the fingers and a history of chronic respiratory infection.[15] Extensive bronchiectasis may be present, with profuse purulent sputum. In other patients, the syndrome of insufficiency of pancreatic enzyme secretion dominates, with poor weight gain despite a voracious appetite, a protuberant abdomen, lack of subcutaneous fat, poor muscle tone and three to six pale, bulky, foul, often greasy stools per day.[21] There may be signs of deficiency of fat-soluble vitamins, such as bleeding and bone pain due to demineralization of bones. If chronic pulmonary disease is also present, the syndrome is even more characteristic. Juvenile-onset diabetes that is rather easily controlled may bring the patient to the physician. Ketoacidosis, retinopathy, neuropathy and nephropathy are usually absent. Recurrent abdominal pain and palpable abdominal masses may be the presenting complaints. The pain is intermittent and the masses represent soft, indentable stool, especially in the right lower quadrant. The pain may vary in severity and location. It may be the result of intestinal obstruction, fecal impaction, bowel distention due to malabsorption or pancreatitis.[10] Meconium ileus is a well known complication of cystic fibrosis in infancy, when the intestine becomes obstructed by masses of meconium. In adolescents and young adults a similar syndrome is known as meconium ileus equivalent. The clinical presentation is that of acute intestinal mechanical obstruction, not explained by other factors such as previous surgery or hernia. It is said to occur in 1 to 10 per cent of patients with cystic fibrosis, and at the Mayo Clinic it accounted for 7 per cent of such patients.[25] In another study, among 70 patients with cystic fibrosis over the age of 25 years, 6 had meconium ileus equivalent.[35]

Hepatomegaly may be a major feature and indicates the development of cirrhosis.[39] Among 693 patients with cystic fibrosis, 15 (2.2 per cent) developed clinical liver disease. In 13, the symptoms were secondary to portal hypertension. Hematemesis or melena was present in 3, resulting from bleeding esophageal varices. Of 116 patients with cystic fibrosis coming to autopsy, 25 had cirrhosis. Typically, the liver is hard, nontender and nodular. Splenomegaly occurs but ascites is uncommon. In men sterility with a nonpalpable vas deferens and small testes may be the presenting syndrome. Of 47 male patients with cystic fibrosis at age 25 and over, all were sterile.[35] In another series of 25 teenagers and adults, there were 3 asymptomatic men, all of whom were sterile.[38] Two of them were found to have aspermia. Women may complain of difficulty of conception, and if this is associated with a history of chest disease, cystic fibrosis should be suspected. Of 23 women with cystic fibrosis over the age of 25, only 8 became pregnant.[35] The menarche was delayed or absent in three of seven women. In a total series of 70 patients, 74 nasal polypectomies had been performed.[35] Any of these symptoms or syndromes in a patient with a family history of cystic fibrosis should suggest the diagnosis. In summary, about 25 per cent of young adults with cystic fibrosis will present with gastrointestinal symptoms, about 30 per cent with respiratory symptoms and about 45 per cent with both.[35] About a third will have had typical symptoms since childhood, but another third will have been asymptomatic until age 13 years.[38]

RISK FACTORS IN THE DIAGNOSIS OF CYSTIC FIBROSIS

Cystic fibrosis is primarily a disease of Caucasians. It is much less frequent in the black population of the United States and almost never occurs in Orientals. There is suggestive evidence of clustering of certain clinical features of cystic fibrosis, e.g., meconium ileus, within families. The severity of the disease may also show clustering within families. Marriage between carriers of the gene for cystic fibrosis is estimated to occur once in every 400 marriages. Consanguinity does not appear to increase the incidence of cystic fibrosis.[6]

LABORATORY DIAGNOSIS OF CYSTIC FIBROSIS

The definitive diagnosis of cystic fibrosis is made by a sweat test demonstrating a chloride or sodium concentration of greater than 50 mEq/L. A quantitative pilocarpine iontophoresis sweat test is more reliable than other methods. Using such a procedure and repeating positive or equivocal tests at least once, the results in 62 patients who had been tested previously were examined. Of 33 patients with previously positive tests, 25 were found to have negative results, and of 29 patients with previously negative tests, 2 were found to have positive results. In only four patients in whom the quantitative test had been done first did the final result differ. It should be noted that adrenal insufficiency, ectodermal dysplasia, nephrogenic diabetes insipidus, hypothyroidism and mucopolysaccharidoses may also produce elevated sodium and chloride values.[31] The greatest source of error comes from a very thin layer of sweat: evaporation can be a problem. The sweat can be collected under an impervious film for 3 minutes before the measurements are made.[3] There is no difference in the sweat electrolyte concentrations between groups 1 to 25 and 25 to 40 years of age.[35]

The secretin-pancreozymin test (see Chapter 3) can be applied to patients with suspected cystic fibrosis. Among 176 patients with cystic fibrosis, 13 had no symptoms of exocrine pancreatic insufficiency or steatorrhea but their stool fat levels were greater than 5 gm/day. Ten of these patients were given 2 units of CCK followed in 20 minutes by 2 units of secretin per kilogram. Duodenal content was collected in 5- to 20-minute samples. All had low volumes and low bicarbonate outputs. Enzyme outputs were variable but the mean did not differ significantly from that of normal subjects,[16-18] while concentrations were high. Compared to noncystic controls, the volume was 0.8 ml/kg/50 min vs. 3.9 ml/kg/50 min, the bicarbonate output was 0.001 to 0.025 mEq/50 min vs. 0.001 to 0.19 mEq/50 min, and bicarbonate concentration was 3.6 to 23.5 mEq/L vs. 49.0 mEq/L.

Results of the glucose tolerance test can be expected to be diabetic in type in about 40 per cent of patients with cystic fibrosis (42 per cent of 31 patients).[19] Serum insulin concentrations were low but rose in response to glucagon or tolbutamide. Overt clinical diabetes was noted in only 7 of 1300 patients with cystic fibrosis.[29] A positive family history of diabetes was obtained in 60 (23 per cent) of 212 patients studied in detail. Glucose tolerance tests were abnormal in 3 of 15 patients selected because of a positive family history of diabetes, whereas glucose tolerance was abnormal in 2 of 15 unselected patients.

In patients presenting with meconium ileus equivalent, the appearance on a survey x-ray film of the abdomen is consistent with mechanical small bowel obstruction.[25, 37] In one study, fecal masses were seen in the right colon in all of 13 patients studied by barium enemas. In 3 the mass was due to intussusception. Esophageal varices can be demonstrated by endoscopy or barium study in patients with portal hypertension. Liver tests are characteristic in those patients with cirrhosis and portal hypertension.[40] The gallbladder was found to be small and shrunken on oral cholecystography in 9 of 17 patients.[11] In another study of 66 subjects with cystic fibrosis, the gallbladder was not visualized on oral cholecystography in 22 patients, and calculi were seen in 3. After intravenous cholangiography a normal ductal system was seen in 6 and a calculus in 1, and the ducts were not visualized in 8 patients.[20]

DIAGNOSIS AND DIFFERENTIAL DIAGNOSIS OF CYSTIC FIBROSIS

The homozygous individual for the gene involved in cystic fibrosis presents in the way described above. Unfortunately there is no satisfactory method of detecting heterozygotes. If the characteristic history is present from childhood and there are siblings with the disease, the diagnosis becomes relatively easy. It is the patients presenting with intestinal obstruction, bleeding esophageal varices, enlarged liver or sterility in the absence of pulmonary symptoms who are most likely to be overlooked. The incidence of cystic fibrosis seems to be reduced in blacks.[34] The diagnosis can be made on the basis of histopathologic changes in the appendix at appendectomy when the mucosa shows increased numbers of goblet cells distended with mucus and wide, gaping intestinal crypts filled with mucus.[34] One series of 14 patients with recurrent abdominal pain had laparotomies and appendectomies with a subsequent diagnosis of cystic fibrosis.

In the series of 70 patients with cystic fibrosis who were over 25 years of age, incorrect previous diagnoses included celiac disease in 15 patients, bronchiectasis in 6, asthma in 5, tuberculosis in 3, histoplasmosis in 1 and delayed sexual maturity in 2.[35] Pancreatic exocrine deficiency due to cystic fibrosis must be differentiated from Shwachman's syndrome (pancreatic insufficiency and neutropenia) and the rare enterokinase deficiency, in which the response to secretin and CCK is usually depressed to a lesser degree and the prognosis is more favorable. Childhood cirrhosis must be differentiated from the biliary cirrhosis of cystic fibrosis.

THE COURSE OF CYSTIC FIBROSIS IN ADOLESCENTS AND YOUNG ADULTS

On the basis of current survival data, it has been predicted that a 15-year-old patient with cystic fibrosis has a life expectancy of 11 years.[42] A projection was made for the 7000 to 54,000 patients with cystic fibrosis in the United States. About 10 per cent of the present cystic fibrosis population are over 25 years of age. The most common complication in this group was pulmonary infection, with cough and hemoptysis in most and pneumothorax in 10 per cent. The most common gastrointestinal complication was fecal impaction, in 17 per cent of 70 patients.[35] Table 5–1 shows additional gastrointestinal complications in the same group of patients. Pancreatitis can occur with hyperamylasemia. In a series of 85 patients, 10 patients over 15 years of age had a history of rectal prolapse, but prolapse after 5 years of age is rare.[22] Patients with portal hypertension who survive an initial variceal bleed are candidates for portal-systemic shunts. Encephalopathy does not seem to occur.[38] The prognosis for survival in cystic fibrosis into adult life is better for males: 47 male to 23 female patients in the group over 25 years of age, and 8 to 4 among patients with symptoms beginning after age 13.[38]

TREATMENT OF CYSTIC FIBROSIS

No curative treatment exists. Pulmonary infections must be treated early and vigorously with antibiotics and pulmonary toilet. Pancre-

*TABLE 5–1. GASTROINTESTINAL COMPLICATIONS**

Fecal impaction	12
Rectal prolapse	5
Rectal bleeding (Vit. K deficiency)	1
Cirrhosis and portal hypertension	2
Intermittent jaundice	2
Diabetes	
Clinical	6
Chemical (47 pts. tested)	11
Recurrent pancreatitis	2
Duodenal ulcer	
elsewhere	3
not confirmed	
Appendicitis	8

From Shwachman, H., Kowalski, M., and Khaw, K-T: Cystic fibrosis: A new outlook. Medicine 56:141, 1977.

atic insufficiency should be treated with eight tablets with each meal of an effective nonenteric-coated pancreatic supplement (see Treatment of Chronic Pancreatitis, Chapter 3). Patients with cirrhosis and portal hypertension who bleed from esophageal varices or have severe hypersplenism are candidates for portal-systemic shunts. Portacaval or splenorenal shunts may be done. In a series of five patients, only one showed progression of liver disease. Only one patient bled again. Two patients died of severe pulmonary disease after 8 years, and three were still alive.[39] In patients with meconium ileus equivalent Gastrografin enemas may be tried initially, but laparotomy may be necessary.[25] In a series of 12 patients, 10 responded to a barium enema, correction of fluid and electrolyte disturbances and pancreatic enzyme supplements.

EPIDEMIOLOGY OF CYSTIC FIBROSIS

The disease occurs in between 1 in 1500 and 1 in 4000 live births.[30, 42] It is uncommon in American blacks and almost unheard of in Orientals. One of every 20 persons, or about 10 million people, are estimated to be carriers of the gene for cystic fibrosis in the United States. Marriage between carriers occurs about once in every 400 marriages. Heterozygote reproduction or survival advantage, or both, that is operative now or was in the past or a genetic drift may account for the high incidence of cystic fibrosis. Epidemiologic studies are handicapped badly by a lack of ability to detect heterozygotes.[6]

PATHOPHYSIOLOGY OF CYSTIC FIBROSIS

This has been studied in cells in vitro and in intact organs. Cultivated fibroblasts from patients with cystic fibrosis show an increased size and number of lysosomes.[1] Metachromatic staining material has been noted in vacuoles or vesicles of cultured cells from patients with cystic fibrosis,[7] but this cannot be used to detect cystic fibrosis in cells in amniotic fluid.[26] The erythrocyte membrane ATPase in patients with cystic fibrosis appears to be normal, but plasma from patients with cystic fibrosis reduces the ATPase activity of normal erythrocytes.[4] The only factor in cystic fibrosis that seems to be related to the pathophysiology is the sodium reabsorption–inhibiting factor acting on sweat glands.[9] The basic defect in cystic fibrosis is unknown. A variety of poorly documented factors inhibit mucociliary function and the reabsorption of sodium in rat parotid and human sweat glands. Mucous glycoproteins demonstrate quantitative abnormalities, but no specific qualitative change in a single glycoprotein has been found. Obstruction of ducts into which mucous secretions are discharged occurs in all patients with cystic fibrosis and is responsible for many of the pathologic features of the disease.[5]

The ratio of spermidine to spermine (polyamines) in the whole blood of patients with cystic fibrosis and heterozygotes is increased, but the biologic significance of this observation is not known.[5] Diminished arginine esterase activity in saliva and plasma of homozygotes has been demonstrated.

Abnormal binding to trypsin of alpha 2-macroglobulin from homozygotes and heterozygotes has been reported. This may be related to deficient proteolytic activity.[5]

Saliva from the minor salivary and parotid glands is abnormal in cystic fibrosis. The sodium concentration is higher than it is in normal subjects.[46] There is fluctuation from day to day in the sodium concentration of parotid saliva from patients with cystic fibrosis; this is found with both unstimulated and stimulated saliva.[12] One group of investigators has found hypersecretion of zymogen granules in the submandibular saliva of patients with cystic fibrosis as well as increased concentrations of calcium, protein and amylase.[2] The saliva was relatively turbid.

There is no evidence of abnormalities of the immune systems in cystic fibrosis. The glucose intolerance appears to be due to "strangulation" of the islets by fibrosis rather than coexistent diabetes mellitus or beta cell loss.[19] The release of insulin into the blood in response to glucose is reduced, and release of both insulin and glucagon in response to arginine is reduced.[6]

There is no evidence of qualitatively abnormal adrenergic responses of the sweat glands.[13] There is also, in patients with cystic fibrosis, a reduced requirement for insulin to dispose of a glucose load and intact glucose tolerance. This suggests increased sensitivity to insulin in the peripheral tissues.

Abnormalities in the intestinal mucosa of patients with cystic fibrosis with and without meconium ileus showed no correlation with the severity of histopathologic changes of the pancreatic disease.[41] However, meconium ileus occurred in patients with intestinal glands filled with mucus. In seven of nine it was a severe degree of change, whereas none of 14 patients without meconium ileus showed comparable changes. The rectal mucosa showed large crypt lumina and, in the epithelial cells, lipid-like droplets that increased during organ culture.[27] Medium chain length triglycerides reduced the steatorrhea of children with cystic fibrosis.[23] Some patients with cystic fibrosis and malabsorption fail to respond to exogenous enzyme therapy. The nature of the absorptive defect is unknown.

Of 116 patients with cystic fibrosis coming to autopsy, 25 had cirrhosis (22 per cent);[8] of these, 6 had multilobular cirrhosis. The earliest lesion was focal biliary cirrhosis with concretions representing inspissated secretion. Cirrhosis with portal hypertension occurred in 7 patients. Patients with cystic fibrosis represented 16 per cent of 57 patients with cirrhosis autopsied at a large children's hospital.[6] The earliest liver changes consist of dilated and proliferating bile ducts in the portal triad secondary to excessive mucus accumulation.

Recently there has been much interest in bile acid metabolism in cystic fibrosis, although the clinical significance is controversial. Fecal bile acids were found to be increased in patients with cystic fibrosis (743 compared to 110 in controls).[45] Excretion was markedly increased when pancreatic enzyme supplements were withdrawn. Patients with cystic fibrosis and liver disease had lower fecal bile acid excretion. The younger patients had higher bile acid outputs.[14] Excessive loss of bile acids occurred only in patients with steatorrhea, although sodium bicarbonate reduced steatorrhea but not fecal loss of bile acids.[44] Bile was found to be lithogenic in its composition of lipids in 26 patients with cystic fibrosis, comparable to that in adults with cholesterol gallstones. Treatment with pancreatic supplements restored bile lipids to normal.[32] Patients with cystic fibrosis excreted smaller amounts of bile acids in breath tests than normal subjects both with and without pancreatic supplements, but the differences were small.[28] It may be that bile acids bind to maldigested proteins, fiber or carbohydrate.[43] The gallbladder has been shown to be approximately half of normal size in about half the patients with cystic fibrosis.[33] Microgallbladder occurred more often in the patients in the 7- to 23-year age group. One patient had asymptomatic gallstones in the gallbladder, and a second may have had symptomatic gallstones. Among 41 patients, the gallbladder was visualized in 22, by oral cholecystography in 17 and intravenous cholangiography in 5.[33] In summary, fecal bile acid excretion is increased in cystic fibrosis, possibly because of binding to undigested protein and carbohydrate. Bile becomes lithogenic, and the incidence of gallstones may increase.

ANIMAL MODELS OF CYSTIC FIBROSIS

There are no satisfactory animal models of cystic fibrosis of the pancreas.

ETIOLOGY OF CYSTIC FIBROSIS

Cystic fibrosis is the most common lethal genetic disease in Caucasian children in the United States. It is generally thought to be transmitted by autosomal recessive inheritance involving a single gene. It has been suggested that the defective gene is localized to the short arm of chromosome number 5, on the basis of observations in a child with both cystic fibrosis and the cri-du-chat syndrome who was found to have deletion of about a third of the short arm of this chromosome.[36]

Heterogeneity of the disorder is to be expected, by analogy with other genetic diseases. Both family and laboratory data in cystic fibrosis are suggestive. Unfortunately, insufficient data are available to test the possibilities of genetic heterogeneity, mutant genes at different loci or allelic variation at a single locus. It is surprising that there has been no study of concordance of cystic fibrosis in twins.[6]

SCREENING FOR CYSTIC FIBROSIS

The quantitative sweat electrolyte test is probably too complex and costly in time and effort for a screening test, but it is possible that a chloride electrode or a conductivity method might be suitable.[11] There is no screening method for heterozygotes.

PREVENTION OF CYSTIC FIBROSIS

There is no satisfactory method of detecting heterozygotes and no intrauterine technique for detecting cystic fibrosis, and so prevention is limited to genetic counseling to prevent recurrence of cystic fibrosis in families already having one affected child.[6] Its effectiveness in unknown. The latest in a series of attempts to identify heterozygotes involves detection of a lectin-like factor in the serum that agglutinates mouse red blood cells. A preliminary report found positive results in 100 per cent of 20 patients with cystic fibrosis and in 60 parents of children with cystic fibrosis but in only 3.75 per cent of 400 mixed controls.[24]

REFERENCES

1. Bartman, J., Wiesmann, U., and Blanc, W. A.: Ultrastructure of cultivated fibroblasts in cystic fibrosis of the pancreas. J. Pediat. 76:430–437, 1970
2. Blomfield, J., Duscalu, J., Van Lenneys, E. W., and Brown, J. M.: Hypersecretion of zymogen granules in the pathogenesis of cystic fibrosis. Gut 14:558–565, 1973
3. Bray, B. I., Clark, G. C. F., Moody, G. J., and Thomas, J. D. R.: Sweat testing for cystic fibrosis. Errors associated with the in-situ sweat test using chloride ion selective electrodes. Clin. Chim. Acta 80:333–338, 1977
4. Cole, C. H., and Dirks, J. H.: Changes in erythrocyte membrane ATPase in patients with cystic fibrosis of the pancreas. Pediat. Res. 6:616–621, 1972
5. Cystic Fibrosis: A Disease in Search of Ideas. Basic Sciences, Vol. 1. Bethesda, Md., U.S. Dept. HEW, Public Health Service, N.I.H., 1979, pp. 1–22
6. Cystic Fibrosis: A Disease in Search of Ideas. Clinical Sciences, Vol., 2. Bethesda, Md., U.S. Dept. HEW, Public Health Service, N.I.H., 1979, pp. 1–41

7. Danes, B. S., and Bearn, A. G.: A genetic cell marker in cystic fibrosis. Lancet 1:1061–1063, 1968
8. di Sant' Agnese, P. A., and Blanc, W. A.: A destructive type of biliary cirrhosis of the liver associated with cystic fibrosis of the pancreas. Pediatrics 18:387–395, 1956
9. di Sant' Agnese, P. A., and Davis, P. B.: Research in cystic fibrosis. New Eng. J. Med. 295:481–485, 534–541, 597–602, 1976
10. di Sant' Agnese, P. A., and Lepore, M. J.: Involvement of abdominal organs in cystic fibrosis of the pancreas. Gastroenterology 40:64–74, 1961
11. Feigelson, J., Pecau, Y., and Sauvegrain, J.: Liver function studies and biliary tract investigations in mucoviscidosis. Acta Pediat. Scand. 59:539–544, 1970
12. Fritz, M. E., Caplan, D. B., Leever, D., and Levitt, J.: Composition of parotid saliva on different days in patients with cystic fibrosis. Am. J. Dis. Child. 123:116–117, 1972
13. Gibson, L. E.: The effect of adrenergic stimulation upon sweating in normal children and cystic fibrosis patients. Pediatrics 48:458–464, 1968
14. Goodchild, M. D., Murphy, G. M., Howell, A. M., Nutter, S. A., and Anderson, C. M.: Aspects of bile acid metabolism in cystic fibrosis. Arch. Dis. Child. 50:769–778, 1975
15. Gracey, M.: Cystic fibrosis. *In* Paediatric Gastroenterology, edited by C. M. Anderson and V. Burke. Oxford, Blackwell Scientific Publications, 1975, pp. 329–359
16. Hadorn, P.: The exocrine pancreas. *In* Paediatric Gastroenterology, edited by C. M. Anderson and V. Burke. Oxford, Blackwell Scientific Publications, 1975, pp. 289–327
17. Hadorn, B., Johansen, P. G., and Anderson, C. M.: Pancreozymin-secretin test for exocrine pancreatic function in cystic fibrosis and the significance of the result for the pathogenesis of the disease. Canad. Med. Assoc. J. 98:377–385, 1968
18. Hadorn, B., Zoppi, G., Shmerling, D. H., Prader, A., McIntire, L., and Anderson, C. M.: Quantitative assessment of exocrine pancreatic function in infants and children. J. Pediat. 73:39–50, 1968
19. Handwerger, S., Roth, J., Gorden, P., di Sant' Agnese, P., Carpenter, D. F., and Peter, G.: Glucose intolerance in cystic fibrosis. New Eng. J. Med. 281:451–461, 1969
20. Isenberg, J. N., L'Heureux, P. R., Warnick, W. J., and Sharp, H. L.: Clinical observations on the biliary system in cystic fibrosis. Am. J. Gastroenterol. 65:134–141, 1976
21. Kopel, F. B.: Gastrointestinal manifestations of cystic fibrosis. Gastroenterology 62:483–492, 1972
22. Kulczycki, L. L., and Shwachman, H.: Studies in cystic fibrosis of the pancreas: Occurrence of rectal prolapse. New Eng. J. Med. 259:409–412, 1958
23. Kuo, P. T., and Huang, N. N.: The effect of MCT upon fat absorption and plasma lipid and depot fat of children with cystic fibrosis of the pancreas. J. Clin. Invest. 44:1924–1933, 1965
24. Lieberman, J., Costea, N., Jakulis, V., and Kaneschiro, W.: Detection of a lectin in the blood of cystic fibrosis: Homozygotes and heterozygotes. Clin. Res. 27:507A, 1979
25. Matseshe, J. W., Go. V. L. W., and DiMagno, E. P.: Meconium ileus equivalent complicating cystic fibrosis in postneonatal children and young adults: Report of 12 cases. Gastroenterology 72:732–736, 1977
26. Nadler, H. L., Swae, M. A., Wodnicki, J. M., and O'Flynn, M. E.: Cultivated amniotic-fluid cells and fibroblasts derived from families with cystic fibrosis. Lancet 2:84, 1969
27. Neutra, M. R., and Trier, J. S.: Rectal mucosa in cystic fibrosis. Gastroenterology 75:701–710, 1978
28. Roller, R. J., and Kern, F.: Minimal bile acid malabsorption and normal bile acid breath tests in cystic fibrosis and acquired pancreatic insufficiency. Gastroenterology 72:661–665, 1977
29. Rosan, R. C., Shwachman, H., and Kulczycki, L. L.: Diabetes mellitus and cystic fibrosis of pancreas: Laboratory and clinical observations. Am. J. Dis. Child. 104:625–634, 1962

30. Rosenlund, M. L., and Lustig, H. S.: Young adults with cystic fibrosis. Ann. Intern. Med. 78:959–961, 1973

31. Rosenstein, B. J., Langbaum, T. S., Gordes, E., and Bruislow, S. W.: Cystic fibrosis: Problems encountered with sweat testing. J.A.M.A. 240:1987–1988, 1978

32. Rovsing, H., and Sloth, K.: Micro-gallbladder and biliary calculi in mucoviscidosis. Acta Radiol. 14:588–592, 1974

33. Roy, C. C., Weber, A. M., Morin, C. L., Combes, J. C., Nussle, D., Megevand, A., and Lasalle, R.: Lithogenic bile in cystic fibrosis: Effect of pancreatic enzymes. New Eng. J. Med. 297:1301–1305, 1977

34. Shwachman, H., and Holsclaw, D.: Examination of the appendix at laparotomy as a diagnostic clue in cystic fibrosis. New Eng. J. Med. 286:1300–1301, 1972

35. Shwachman, H., Kowalski, M., and Khaw, K-T.: Cystic fibrosis: A new outlook. Medicine 56:129–149, 1977

36. Smith, D. W., Docter, J. M., Ferrier, P. E., Frias, J. L., and Spock, A.: Possible localization of the gene for cystic fibrosis of the pancreas to the short arm of chromosome 5. Lancet 2:309–312, 1968

37. Snyder, W. H., Gwinn, J. L., Landing, B. H., and Asay, L. D.: Fecal retention in children with cystic fibrosis. Pediatrics 34:72–77, 1964

38. Stern, R. C., Boat, T. F., Doershuk, C. F., Tucker, A. S., Miller, R. B., and Matthews, L. W.: Cystic fibrosis diagnosed after age 13. Ann. Intern. Med. 87:188–191, 1977

39. Stern, R. C., Stevens, D. P., Boat, T. F., Doershak, C. F., Izant, R. J., Jr., and Matthews, L. W.: Symptomatic hepatic disease in cystic fibrosis: Incidence, course and outcome of portal systemic shunting. Gastroenterology 70:645–649, 1976

40. Swift, P. N.: Cystic fibrosis of the pancreas and biliary cirrhosis. Proc. Roy. Soc. Med. 56:923–924, 1963

41. Thomaidis, T. S., and Arey, J. B.: Intestinal lesions in cystic fibrosis of the pancreas. J. Pediat. 63:444–453, 1963

42. Warwick, W. J., and Pogue, R. E.: Cystic fibrosis: An expanding challenge for internal medicine. J.A.M.A. 238:2159–2162, 1977

43. Watkins, J. B., Lercyak, A. M., Szczepanik, P., and Klein, P. D.: Bile salt kinetics in cystic fibrosis: Influence of pancreatic enzyme replacement. Gastroenterology 73:1023–1028, 1977

44. Weber, A. M., Roy, C. C., Chartrand, L., Lepage, G., Dufour, O. L., Morin, C. L., and Lasalle, R.: Relationship between bile acid malabsorption and pancreatic insufficiency in cystic fibrosis. Gut 17:295–299, 1976

45. Weber, A. M., Roy, C. C., Morin, C. L., and Lasalle, R.: Malabsorption of bile acids in children with cystic fibrosis. New Engl. J. Med. 289:1001–1005, 1973

46. Wiesmann, U. N., Boat, T. F., and di Sant' Agnese, P. A.: Sodium concentration in unstimulated parotid saliva and on oral mucosa in normal subjects and in patients with cystic fibrosis. J. Pediat. 76:444–448, 1970

SECTION II

BASIC CONSIDERATIONS

In this section, I present a summary of our current knowledge of the physiology of the pancreas. The reader may wish to refer to the sections dealing with pathophysiology of the individual diseases for the relevance of these basic considerations to clinical problems.

CHAPTER 6

THE STRUCTURAL BASIS AND PHYSIOLOGY OF EXOCRINE PANCREATIC SECRETION

THE STRUCTURAL BASIS OF PANCREATIC EXOCRINE SECRETION

The pancreas is a relatively inaccessible organ in man. Until recently, the structure of the exocrine ducts could be seen only after injection of radiopaque material into the sphincter of Oddi, and the pancreatic ducts only at the time of laparotomy. Endoscopic retrograde cholangiopancreatography (ERCP) has changed all this, and we have since learned to identify the normal pattern of branching of the pancreatic ducts and their relation to the acini. As will be noted later, the acinar cells bordering the terminal acini are the source of the enzymes in pancreatic exocrine secretion.[20] The source of fluid and electrolyte is controversial but it is likely that much of the fluid and bicarbonate is added by the ducts. This "two-component" theory is a feature of explanations of the varying composition of secretion in tubulo-alveolar glands elsewhere in the body. Figure 6–1 shows a roentgenogram of the human pancreas in vitro after injection of barium through the sphincter of Oddi. The ductal structures and acini are well displayed.[4]

The structure of a pancreatic acinar cell as seen with the electron microscope is shown in Figure 6–2. It is thought that each pancreatic zymogen granule contains nearly all the enzymes and proenzymes of pancreatic juice. Recent evidence suggests that the enzyme complement of acinar cells near the islets of Langerhans (peri-insular cells)

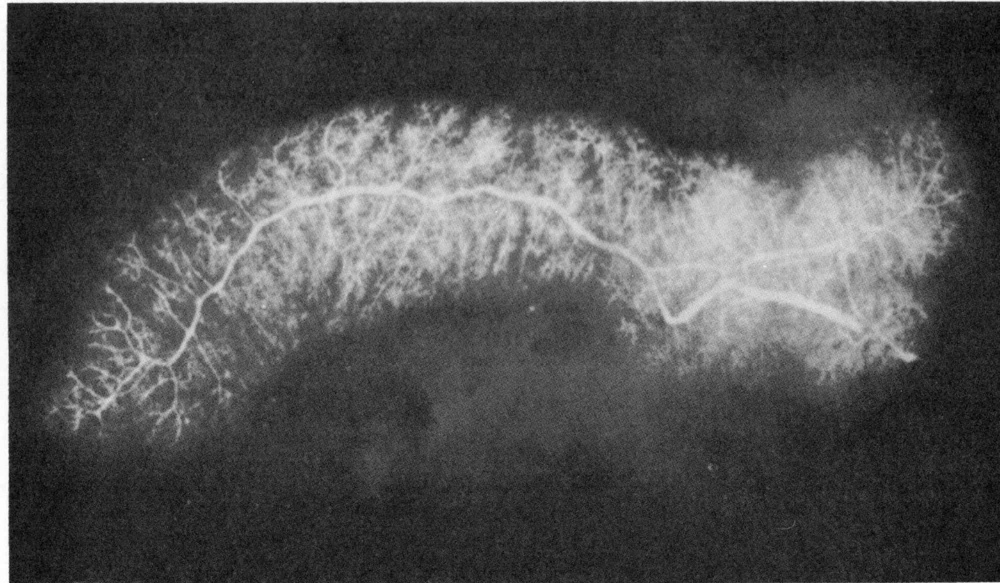

Figure 6–1.   Roentgenogram of human pancreas after removal from the body and filling of the ducts with a solution of barium injected through the sphincter of Oddi. Note gradual tapering in the size of the ducts and filling of the terminal ducts and acini. (From Kreel, L., Sandin, B., and Slavin, G.: Pancreatic morphology. A combined radiological and pathological study. Clin. Radiol. 24:154–161, 1973.)

may have a different composition of pancreatic enzymes from other acinar cells. According to Palade, proenzymes are synthesized on the rough endoplasmic reticulum, enter the cisternae, and pass on to the Golgi apparatus, where they are enclosed in an enveloping membrane — the zymogen granule. These granules then traverse the cell cytoplasm and fuse with the apical cell membrane and extrude their contents into the lumen (exocytosis).[4] Alternatives to this theory will be considered later.

THE PHYSIOLOGY OF EXOCRINE PANCREATIC SECRETION

Our knowledge of the mechanisms and control of pancreatic secretion has advanced substantially because of the availability of new techniques and the purification and synthesis of peptides acting on the pancreas. It is now possible to obtain from guinea pig or rat isolated dispersed pancreatic acinar cells that will respond to stimulants by releasing pancreatic enzymes, usually amylase, into the medium.[2, 17] In current terminology this is conceived as an interaction

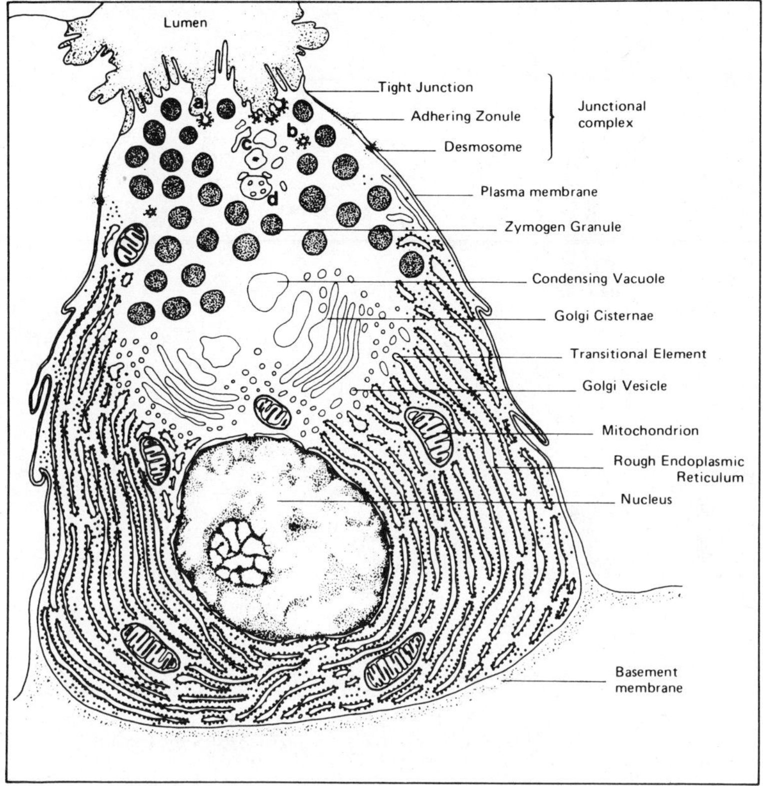

Figure 6–2. Diagram of a pancreatic acinar cell. The sequence of events (*a–d*) illustrated in the apical zone of the cell represents the features of secretion of enzymatic protein: *a* = caveolus; *b* = coated vesicle; *c* = endocytotic vesicle; and *d* = multivesicle body. (From Case, R. M.: Synthesis, intracellular transport and discharge of exportable proteins in the pancreatic acinar cell and other cells. Proc. Aust. Physiol. Pharmacol. Soc. 9:29–42, 1978.)

between the stimulant molecule and a receptor on the surface of the cell.[6] At least three classes of receptors of likely physiologic significance have been identified: acetylcholine, cholecystokinin (CCK) and secretin receptors. Acetylcholine's effect on amylase release can be blocked by atropine, but this anticholinergic agent has no effect on CCK's release of amylase. The evidence indicates that separate, distinct receptors must exist. Secretin also stimulates amylase release, but there is no evidence for competitive interaction with the other stimulants, again indicating a separate receptor mechanism.

The nature of the binding between stimulant and acinar cell can be studied quantitatively and in general fits well with the physiologic action of the stimulant, although exceptions exist. These studies have permitted further experiments to determine the mechanism of action of the stimulants in causing enzyme secretion. Two distinct mechan-

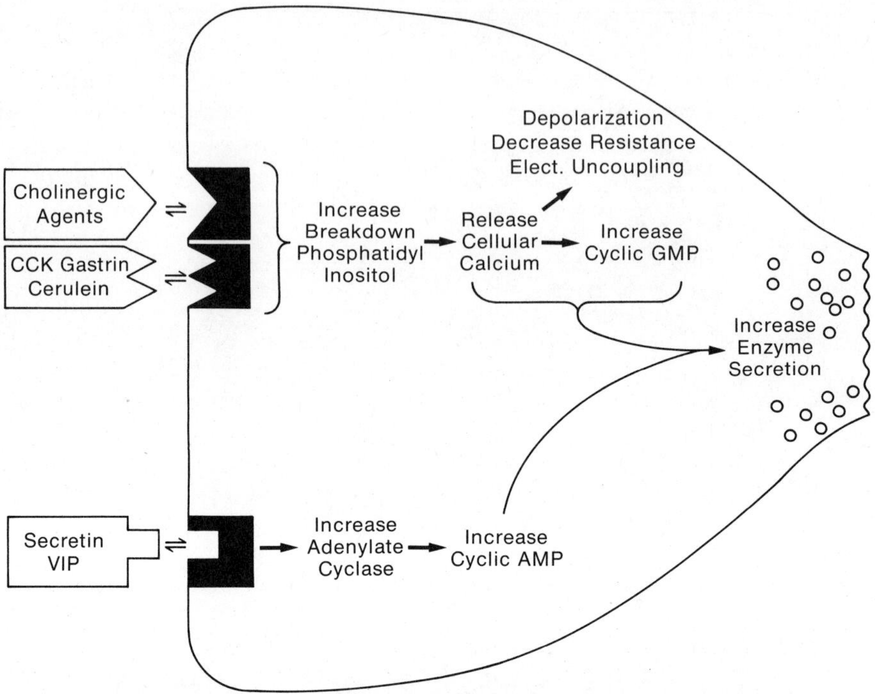

Figure 6–3.   Interaction of acetylcholine and gastrointestinal peptides with pancreatic acinar cells. (Courtesy of Dr. J. D. Gardner, National Institute of Arthritis, Metabolism and Digestive Diseases, Bethesda, Md., 1979.)

isms exist, one characterized by acetylcholine and CCK and the other by secretin. As a result of the interaction of CCK with the cell membrane, calcium is released from an intracellular binding site, and this in some unknown way stimulates intracellular secretory activity. The final step of escape of enzyme from the cell membrane by exocytosis (reverse pinocytosis) is also calcium dependent. Cyclic GMP formation is enhanced, but this is probably an epiphenomenon rather than a necessary step in secretion. Eventually calcium enters the cell to restore intracellular stores.

In the case of secretin, the initial step is the activation of adenyl cyclase in the cell membrane, with an increase in the formation of intracellular cyclic AMP. This in turn results in the activation of protein kinases, which stimulate the secretion of enzymes. Figure 6–3 gives a diagrammatic representation of these events. Experiments with perfused cat pancreas also confirm the role of cyclic AMP in the action of secretin on pancreatic secretion.[15, 16]

It is also known that acetylcholine and CCK partially depolarize pancreatic acinar cells, probably by increasing the cell membrane's permeability to sodium. This phenomenon is not necessarily followed by secretion of enzyme. Atropine again selectively blocks the action of acetylcholine but not that of CCK.[11]

The events occurring within the acinar cell have been studied by radioautography and electron microscopy, with the resulting hypothesis: the enzymatic proteins are synthesized on the rough endoplasmic reticulum (RER) by microsomes.[10] They are then inserted through the membrane into the lumen of the channels in the RER. From here on they are contained within membranes and effectively excluded from the intracellular environment. Within the Golgi apparatus they are packaged within zymogen granules, which then move to the cell surface, where they are extruded by a process of reverse pinocytosis. An implication of this hypothesis is that the complement of enzymes within each granule or group of granules should be similar, and parallel secretion of the pancreatic enzymes should follow. "Nonparallel" secretion does occur in response to certain stimuli and in the process of adaptation to various diets. An alternative hypothesis is that enzymes are able to move across intracellular compartments in response to diffusion gradients.[13] The design of experiments to sharp-

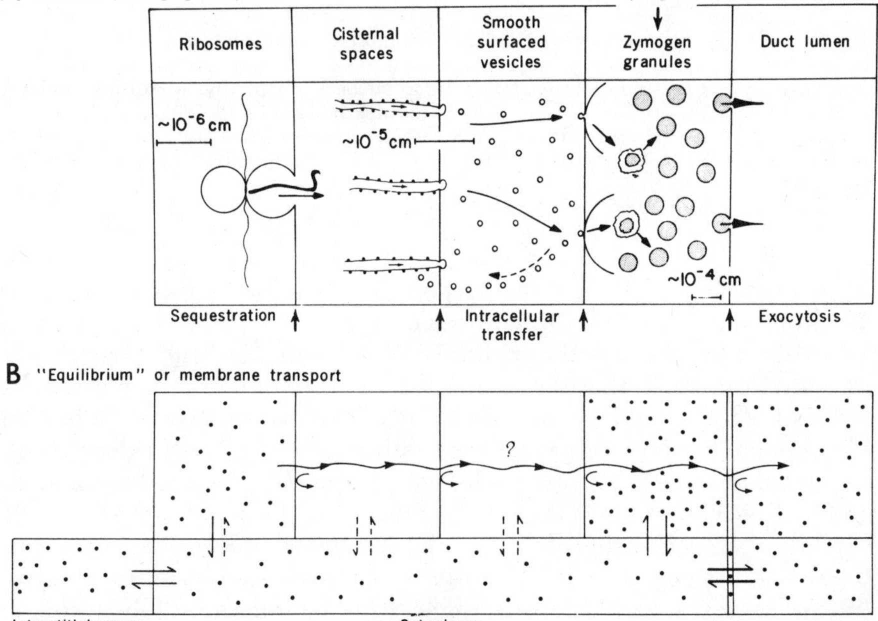

Figure 6–4. Models of secretion of digestive enzymes by the pancreas. *A,* The classic cisternal packaging route of Palade. *B,* An alternative route with equilibration between a number of compartments within the cytoplasm acts as a mixing chamber for enzymes from other pools and as a direct precursor pool for secretion. Dots indicate individual protein molecules in relative density. Wavy lines indicate that a cisternal pathway may also occur. Solid arrows indicate processes for which there is evidence. (From Rothman, S. S.: Protein transport by the pancreas. Science 190:747–753, Nov. 21, 1975. Copyright 1975 by the American Association for the Advancement of Science.)

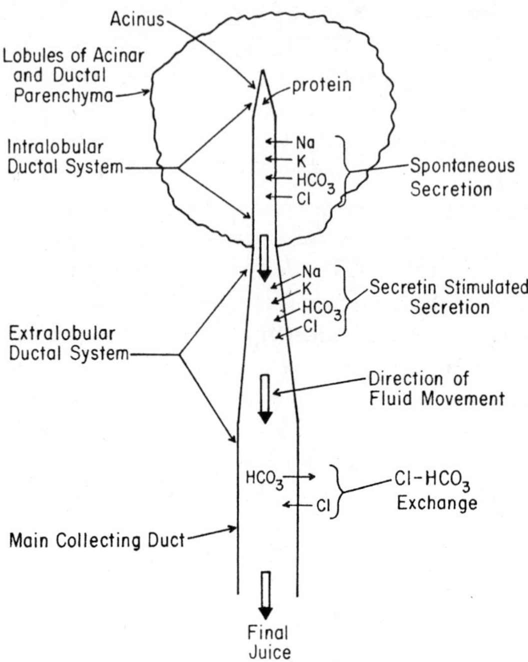

Figure 6–5.   Diagram of pancreatic acinus and duct system ("pancreon"). Sodium bicarbonate is probably also secreted in the acinus. The effects of inhibitors of sodium transport suggest that active transport of sodium occurs proximally. Secretin stimulates a bicarbonate "pump" to add a solution of bicarbonate in the extralobular ducts. (From Swanson, C. H., and Solomon, A. K.: A micropuncture investigation of the whole tissue mechanism of electrolyte secretion by the in vitro rabbit pancreas. J. Gen. Physiol. 62:426, 1973.)

ly distinguish between these hypotheses has been difficult. Figure 6–4 illustrates these two hypotheses.

Micropuncture of the pancreatic ducts in several species has provided evidence that the acinar fluid is rich in chloride but that as the fluid passes down the ducts it becomes relatively richer in bicarbonate, probably as a result of both an active, secretin-dependent bicarbonate pump and an exchange of chloride for bicarbonate, as shown in Figure 6–5.[14] The concentration of bicarbonate in pancreatic secretion depends, therefore, on the length of time the secretion in the ducts is exposed to the chloride-bicarbonate exchange mechanism (rate of secretion) and the level of secretin stimulation of bicarbonate secretion into the ducts. These concepts are important for the interpretation of the secretin test. As the dose of secretin is increased, the volume of pancreatic secretion and bicarbonate concentration increase rapidly in an exponential fashion. With still further increasing doses of secretin, however, the volume continues to increase but the bicarbonate concentration remains constant. Therefore, bicarbonate output is a better indicator of pancreatic secretory capacity than bicarbonate concentration. With prolonged secretin stimulation, bicarbonate concentration may actually fall while output remains constant.

The bicarbonate-secreting capacity of the normal pancreas exceeds the stomach's acid-secreting capacity. Yet, under normal circumstances in man, more acid than bicarbonate is secreted in response to a meal, with a resulting alkaline tide in the urine.

Pancreatic bicarbonate is formed mostly from plasma bicarbonate with a small contribution from endogenous cellular carbon dioxide. It is not clear whether the initial event is transport of H^+ into the cell or the efflux of HCO_3. The net effect is transport of HCO_3 into the lumen and H^+ into the plasma in equal amounts. The pancreatic duct cells are probably the site of bicarbonate secretion.[3]

The relationship between rate of secretion and bicarbonate and chloride concentrations could be explained by acinar-ductular two-component secretion, ion exchange in the ducts or variable cellular transport of sodium, bicarbonate and chloride. It is not possible to choose among these three hypotheses.[9]

The pancreas secretes a large number of proteases — exopeptidases, endopeptidases and phospholipases — all in an inactive form, along with an inhibitory protein as added insurance against intracellular activation and autodigestion. Activation of trypsinogen by enterokinase from the brush borders of small intestinal mucosal surface epithelial cells occurs through the splitting off of a hexapeptide. Once active trypsin is present, an autocatalytic process follows, and the other precursor proteolytic enzymes are converted to active enzymes. Figure 6–6 shows this sequence of events. It is this initial conversion of trypsinogen to trypsin that many students of pancreatic

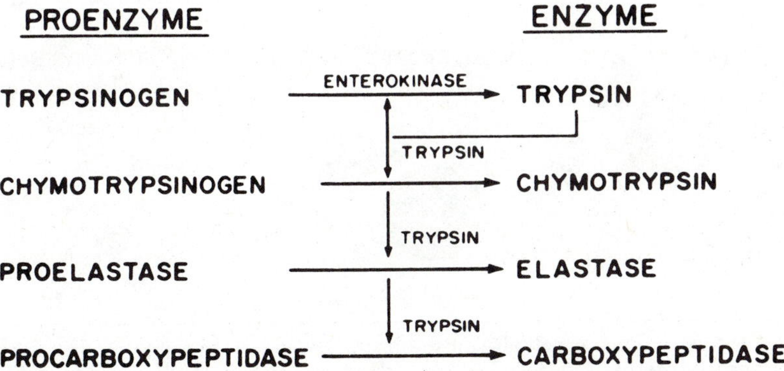

Figure 6–6.   Activation of the proteolytic proteases in the duodenal lumen. (From Gray, G. M., and Cooper, H. L.: Protein digestion and absorption. Gastroenterology 61:536, 1971. © 1971 The Williams & Wilkins Co., Baltimore.)

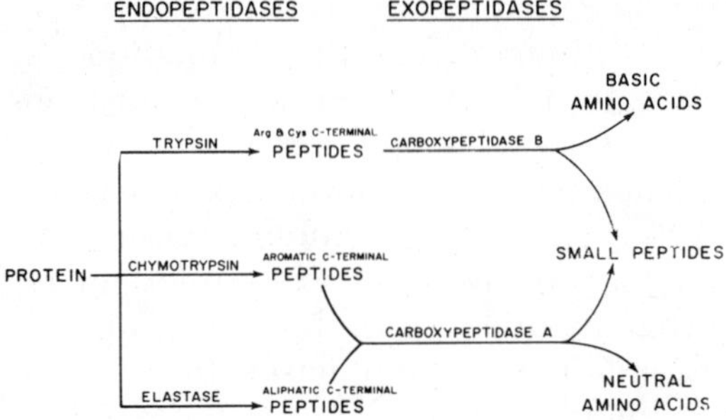

Figure 6–7. Intraduodenal sequential action of pancreatic endopeptidases and exopeptidases on dietary protein. The final products on the right are the substrates that must be handled by the intestinal cell. Arg = arginine; Cys = cysteine. (From Gray, G. M., and Cooper, H. L.: Protein digestion and absorption. Gastroenterology 61:537, 1971. © 1971 The Williams & Wilkins Co., Baltimore.)

disease believe is the first step in the development of acute pancreatitis. The combined action of endopeptidases and exopeptidases leads to the production of amino acids and small peptides in intestinal content, as shown in Figure 6–7.

Pancreatic lipase is present in pancreatic secretion as an active enzyme. In the presence of bile acids, however, lipolysis of triglycerides is inhibited unless another protein, colipase, is present. This molecule binds to the surface of the triglyceride molecule and permits the lipase to attach to it (Fig. 6–8). It also protects lipase against the inhibitory action of bile acids by binding to micelles.

Phospholipase and elastase are of particular interest because their actions simulate most closely the lesions seen in acute pancreatitis: destruction of blood vessel walls (elastase) and cellular necrosis (phospholipase).

It should be noted that the products of the interaction between pancreatic enzymes are monoglycerides, fatty acids and glycerol; maltose, triose, monosaccharides and oligosaccharides, and peptides

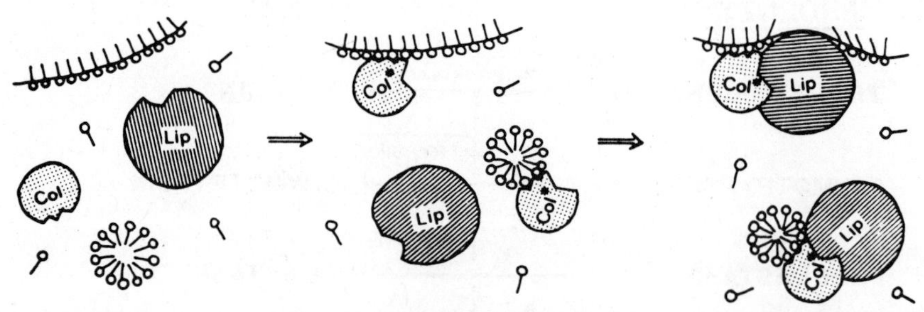

Figure 6–8. Roles of colipase in the fixation of lipase to a hydrophilic interface (micelle or triglyceride interface coated with an amphipath). Col* designates the cofactor form in which a binding site for lipase has been created for adsorption to micelle or interface. (From Desnuelle, P.: The lipase-colipase system. *In* Lipid Absorption: Biochemical and Clinical Aspects, edited by K. Rommel and H. Goebell. MTP Press, Lancaster, England, 1976, p. 32.)

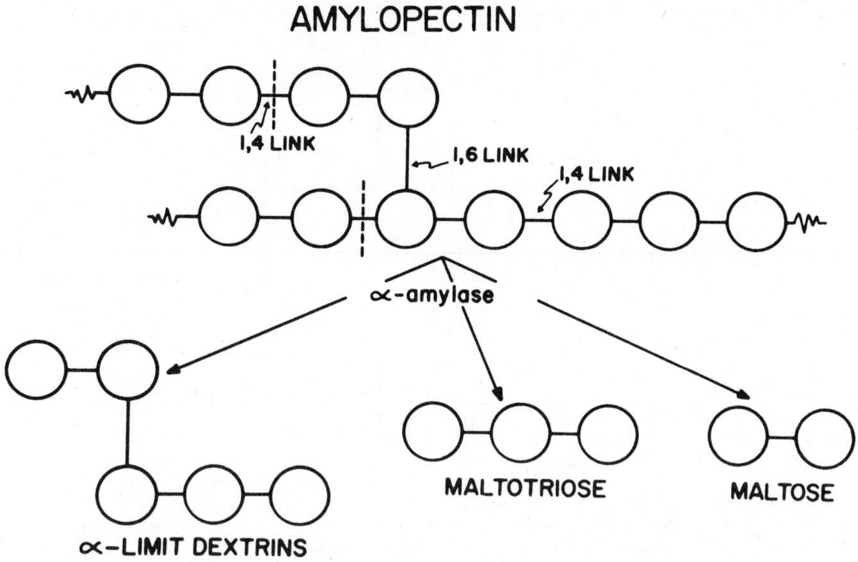

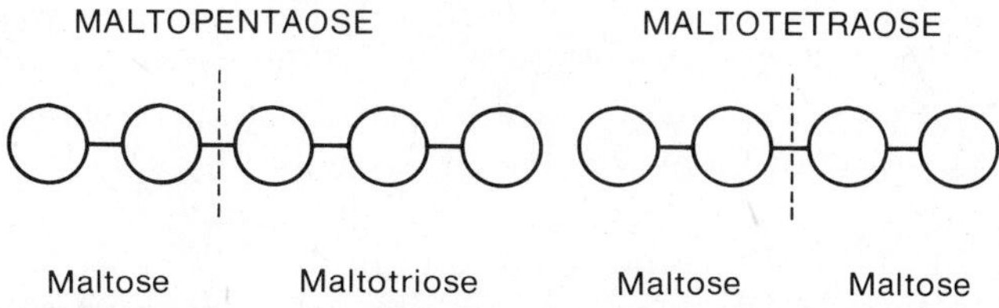

Figure 6–9. Tetra- and pentasaccharide products of amylase digestion. Each circle represents a glucose molecule, and the bridging lines indicate 1,4 α links. Dotted lines are located at sites of amylase action on the interior of the molecule, yielding tri- and disaccharides as the final hydrolytic products. (From Gray, G. M.: Carbohydrate digestion and absorption. Gastroenterology 58:97, 1970.) © 1970 The Williams & Wilkins Co., Baltimore.

and amino acids. Digestion is completed at the brush border membrane of the intestinal mucosal epithelial cells.[1]

The major dietary carbohydrate is starch. This is a combination of amylase, a polymer of linear chains of glucose, and amylopectin, which in addition includes branching points of additional glucose chains. Pancreatic α amylase splits amylase into 2, 3, 4 and 5 glucose chain moleclues (Fig. 6–9). The latter are then split into 2 and 3 glucose chains (maltose and maltotriose), which become the final products of the pancreatic digestion of amylase (Fig. 6–10). In the case of amylopectin, the digestion products include larger molecules such as

Figure 6–10. Final products of amylopectin hydrolysis. A segment of the amylopectin is shown. Each circle represents a glucose unit. The sites of α amylase action are shown by the dotted lines. (From Gray, G. M.: Carbohydrate digestion and absorption. Role of the small intestine. New Eng. J. Med. 292:1225, 1975.)

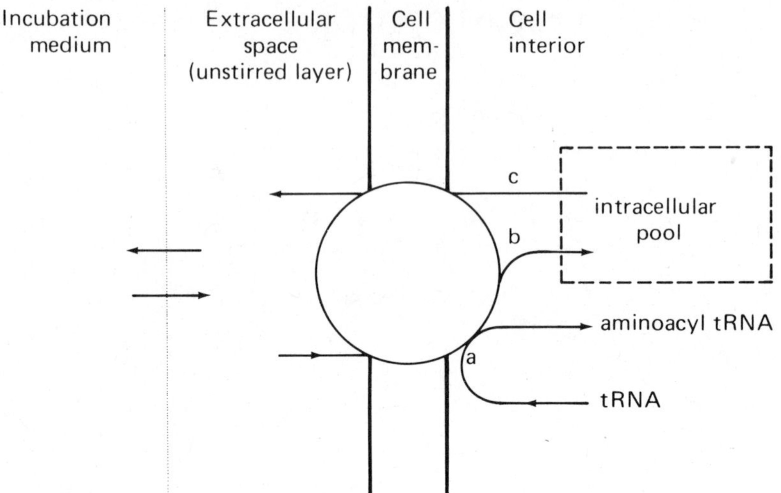

Figure 6–11.   Postulated model for entrance of amino acids into pancreatic acinar cell. Amino acids in the extracellular space are transported into the membrane by an appropriate carrier. A given amino acid may be picked up by an appropriate transfer RNA molecule (tRNA) to form aminoacyl-tRNA (route *a*) and hence be incorporated into protein (see Fig. 6–12). Excess, nonactivated amino acids enter the intracellular pool (route *b*) from which they can exchange with other amino acids in the extracellular fluid (route *c*), probably using the same carrier mechanism. Based on a model by van Venrooij *et al.* (1972). (From Case, R. M.: Synthesis, intracellular transport and discharge of exportable proteins in the pancreatic acinar cell and other cells. Biol. Rev. 53:211–354, 1978. By permission of the Cambridge University Press.)

α limit dextrins (Fig. 6–9). These are added to the maltose and maltotriose in the lumen as a result of the digestion of amylase.

The pancreas is the site of intense protein synthetic activity. Amino acids are actively taken up by pancreatic acinar cells. It appears that some enter an intracellular pool in equilibrium with extracellular fluid and others are picked up by transfer RNA molecules and bound together with messenger RNA to ribosomal subunits to form a functional ribosome where the appropriate amino acids and transfer RNAs (aminoacyl-tRNA), containing complementary base triplets (anticodons), attach sequentially to the ribosome opposite the appropriate codons. A peptide bond is formed between the aminoacyl-tRNA and the lengthening peptide, with simultaneous release of the previously attached transfer RNA (Figs. 6–11 and 6–12). Termination of the polypeptide chain is signaled by special condons in the messenger RNA, and the complete protein and free messenger RNA detach from the ribosome. It is thought that all messenger RNAs that are to be translated on membrane-bound ribosomes contain an initial sequence of codons (purine bases) that produce a unique sequence of amino acids. This sequence, when the peptide emerges from the ribosome, leads to an attachment of the ribosome to the rough endoplasmic reticulum (RER), creating a pore through which the new protein can enter into the cisternae of the RER and begin its journey toward the Golgi apparatus and the formation of zymogen granules (Fig. 6–12).

The use of selenomethionine to scan the pancreas or to label pancreatic enzymes in duodenal content is based upon this sequence of events.

Cell replication rates can be altered by gastrointestinal peptide hormones. This is known as a trophic action of hormones.[8] In animals, both gastrin and CCK increase pancreatic weight and the incorporation of labeled amino acids into protein or tritiated thymidine into DNA and RNA. Combinations of secretin and CCK given over longer periods increase pancreatic weight and pancreatic secretory capacity

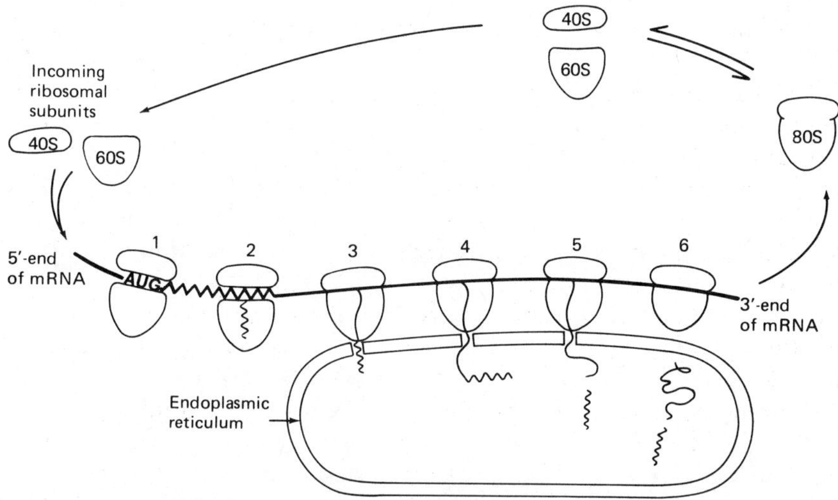

Figure 6–12. Translation and the signal hypothesis. Amino acids are first activated by combination with specific transfer RNA molecules to form aminoacyl-tRNAs. Messenger RNA (mRNA) and a particular aminoacyl-tRNA then bind to the 40S ribosomal subunit and together these combine with a 60S ribosomal subunit to form a functional (80S) ribosome. The sequence of base triplets (codons) in mRNA is decoded by the ribosome. Aminoacyl-tRNAs possessing complementary base triplets (anticodons) sequentially attach to the ribosome opposite appropriate codons. A peptide bond is formed between the incoming aminoacyl-tRNA and the lengthening peptide with simultaneous release of the previously attached, and now vacant, tRNA. Termination of the polypeptide chain is signaled by special codons in mRNA and the complete protein and free mRNA detach from the ribosome. Translation of mRNA by several ribosomes may occur simultaneously so that, during cell fractionation, ribosomes are often isolated as clusters called polyribosomes or polysomes held together by an mRNA strand. Essential features of the signal hypothesis are shown by the zig-zag region in the mRNA strand immediately after the initiation codon AUG (adenine-uridine-guanine) indicating signal codons. The signal sequence of amino acids on the nascent polypeptide chain is indicated by the broken line. (Modified from Case, R. M.: Pancreatic secretion: cellular aspects. *In* Scientific Basis of Gastroenterology, edited by K. G. Wormsley and H. L. Duthie. New York, Churchill Livingstone, 1979, p. 172.)

in response to hormonal stimulation. Trypsin inhibitors fed to animals also increase pancreatic weight, suggesting a feedback regulation between trypsin in the lumen of the gut and the amount of CCK released into the circulation. Confirmation of this awaits a satisfactory CCK radioimmunoassay.

Dietary changes can lead to adaptive changes in the proportion of proteolytic, lipolytic and starch-splitting enzymes secreted. The mechanism of adaptation is unknown.[18]

Under basal resting conditions pancreatic secretion occurs at a very low level. After each meal, however, the pancreas secretes large amounts of both enzymes and bicarbonate.

The purification, isolation and determination of the structure of the major identified gut peptide hormones acting on the pancreas have greatly advanced our knowledge of pancreatic physiology. A sensitive radioimmunoassay for secretin is now available in several laboratories.[19] Although CCK may well prove to be the most important controlling factor in pancreatic enzyme secretion, as well as the phylogenetically oldest of the gastrointestinal peptides, we still have no satisfactory radioimmunoassay for it.[5] The pancreas is well represented as a target for the action of "candidate hormones" in the gut.[7, 12] Radioimmunoassay shows that there is a small rise in serum secretin, usually as periodic brief spikes, that correlates with increases in bicarbonate secretion and rises in intraduodenal pH. Amino acids, especially tryptophan and phenylalanine, in the duodenum and proximal jejunum stimulate the secretion of pancreatic enzymes, although lack of a suitable sensitive radioimmunoassay prevents conclusive demonstration that this is mediated by CCK. The action of fats in stimulating the secretion of both bicarbonate and enzymes may be due to potentiation of secretin and CCK released simultaneously or to the release of currently unknown substances. Since a transplanted pancreas responds qualitatively to a meal in much the same fashion as the intact organ, it was assumed that hormones played the major role in mediating the exocrine pancreatic response to a meal. Recently it has been possible to compare the response to a meal of an intact innervated portion of the pancreas with that of a transplanted portion in conscious dogs. It was shown that the intact pancreas was much more sensitive than the transplant in terms of its secretory response to exogenous CCK-like peptides and to endogenous release of CCK. Furthermore, administration of atropine reduced the responsiveness of the intact pancreas to that of the transplant. These observations suggest that local cholinergic nervous mechanisms play an important role in the normal response to a meal. They suggest a possible explanation for the maldigestion due to impairment of pancreatic secretion that is sometimes seen after truncal vagotomy. Figure 6–13 shows a schema for vagal control of pancreatic enzyme secretion.

Secretin and CCK have been demonstrated in the granules of

DIRECT CHOLINERGIC EFFECTS

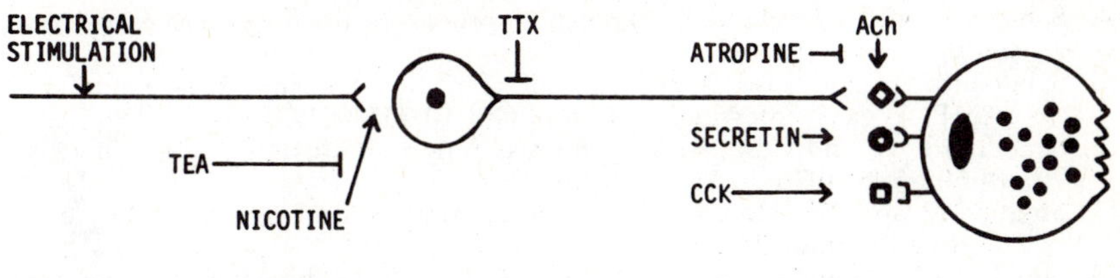

Figure 6–13.   Schematic diagram of evidence favoring direct cholinergic effects on pancreatic secretion. (From Solomon, T., and Grossman, M. I.: Vagal control of pancreatic exocrine secretion. *In* Nerves and the Gut, edited by F. P. Brooks and P. W. Evers. Thorofare, N.J., Charles B. Slack, 1977, p. 123.)

individual endocrine cells of the small intestinal mucosa by immunocytochemistry. Loss of these cells in small intestinal mucosal disease, such as celiac sprue, accounts for decreased pancreatic secretion in response to a meal even though the response to exogenous hormones remains normal.

REFERENCES

1. Brooks, F. P.: Steps in digestion and absorption in the small bowel. *In* Scientific Foundations of Gastroenterology, edited by W. Sircus and A. N. Smith. London, William Heinemann Medical Books, 1980
2. Case, R. M.: Synthesis, intracellular transport and discharge of exportable proteins in the pancreatic acinar cell and other cells. Biol. Rev. 53:211–354, 1978
3. Case, R. M.: Secretory processes in exocrine pancreas. Proc. Aust. Physiol. Pharmacol. Soc. 9:29–42, 1978
4. Case, R. M.: Pancreatic secretion: Cellular aspects. *In* Scientific Basis of Gastroenterology, edited by H. L. Duthie and K. G. Wormsley. Edinburgh, Churchill Livingstone, 1979, pp. 163–198
5. Dockray, G. J.: Molecular evolution of gut hormones. Gastroenterology 72:344–358, 1977
6. Gardner, J. D.: Receptors for gastrointestinal hormones. Gastroenterology 76:202–214, 1979
7. Grossman, M. I.: Candidate hormones of the gut. Gastroenterology 67:730–755, 1974
8. Johnson, L. R.: New aspects of the trophic action of gastrointestinal hormones. Gastroenterology 72:788–792, 1977
9. Makhlouf, G. M., and Blum, A. L.: An assessment of models of pancreatic secretion. Gastroenterology 59:896–908, 1970
10. Palade, G.: Intracellular aspects of the process of protein synthesis. Science 189:347–358, 1975
11. Peterson, O. H.: Electrophysiology of mammalian gland cells. Physiol. Rev. 56:535–577, 1976
12. Rayford, P. L., Miller, T. A., and Thompson, J. C.: Secretin, cholecystokinin and

newer gastrointestinal hormones. New Eng. J. Med. 294:1093–1100, 1157–1164, 1976
13. Rothman, S. S.: Protein transport by the pancreas. Science 190:747–753, 1975
14. Schulz, I., and Ullrich, K. J.: Transport processes in the exocrine pancreas. In press.
15. Scratcherd, T., and Case, R. M.: The role of cyclic adenosine-3′,5′-monophosphate (AMP) in gastrointestinal secretion. Gut 10:951–961, 1969
16. Scratcherd, T., and Case, R. M.: Progress report: Perfusion of the pancreas. Gut 14:592–598, 1973
17. Singh, M., and Webster, P. D.: Neurohumoral control of pancreatic secretion. Gastroenterology 74:294–309, 1978
18. Snook, J. I.: Adaptive and non-adaptive changes in digestive enzyme capacity influencing digestive function. Fed. Proc. 33:88–93, 1974
19. Straus, E.: Radioimmunoassay of gastrointestinal hormones. Gastroenterology 74:141–152, 1978
20. Webster, P. D., Black, O., Mainz, D. L., and Singh, M.: Pancreatic acinar cell metabolism and function. Gastroenterology 73:1434–1449, 1977

INDEX

Numbers followed by "t" refer to tables; numbers
in *italics* refer to illustrations.